500 Fruit Infused Water Recipes

The Freeway to Touch a Healthy Lifestyle

Annie Kate

Contents

Introduction

If you are a person having a healthy lifestyle, or being on the way to get a healthy life, I am sure that the following words I am about to mention will not strange to you. These are "Fruit Infused Water Recipes for Weight Loss"! They are the words regarding as one of the most "HOT" key words through the years. So, **500 Fruit Infused Water Recipes** was born to help you have a list of fruit infused recipes which surely become a best friend in your life every day.

Firstly, I want you to know about the importance of water in our life. As you know, water makes up more than 65% in our body and helps other parts in the body such as Liver and Kidney operated effectively. So, if we do not drink enough water each day, our body will be slow and caught many diseases. How much is enough? Actually, the much you drink, the better you are. But to be exactly, if your weight is 50kg, you need to charge 2 liters of water in your body each day. Thus, let's start your day with a cup of water to charge energy for all work day!

However, many people said that they do not like drinking water, or they cannot drink water all day, so Fruit Infused Drinks were born to make people charge water into their body by another more interesting way because they are more delicious than water, and we can make it with a variety of different ways. In general, Fruit Infused Drinks are healthy beverages with quick and easy methods to make. They are the infusions of water, fruits, herbs, etc. They are also juices, or smoothies. I strongly believe that my book will be very useful to you and surely you will love it.

"500 Fruit Infused Water Recipes" is a collection of 500 QUICK

& EASY Fruit Infused Drink Recipes with Clear Instructions and Real Imagines. It will in include the following parts:

- ✓ *One: Detox Water*
- ✓ *Two: Detox Juice*
- ✓ *Three: Detox Smoothie*
- ✓ *Four: Mocktail Recipes*
- ✓ *Five: Non-alcoholic Punch Recipes*
- ✓ *Six: Tea Recipes*
- ✓ *Seven: More Healthy Drink Recipes*

What about Detox Water for Weight Loss? Detox water is a type of Fruit Infused Water. In fact, the main function of Detox Drinks is getting rid of body toxin. When the toxin is dismissed, the parts in the body are operated better, and from that it will help to Boost Metabolism. That Metabolism is boosted will make our body consume Calories effectively. So, our weight will be decreased. Moreover, drinking more water will make us eat less each meal have the "full" feeling in our stomach. When we recall the word "Detox", we will think about Weight Loss immediately, but there are less people knowing many other benefits of Detox Drink. I will sum up by the following phrases to help you get the other advantages when drinking Detox Drinks: "Healthy Skin, Metabolism Boosting, Productivities Improvement, Energy Boosting, Fights Infections, Risk of Cancel Reducing, Healthy Heart, Stress Releasing."

In addition, after a long time we charge toxin from food, soda, alcohol drinks, others, our body need being detoxed. Fruit Infused Drinks will be the best choice for us at that time. If you want to lose your weight, replace soda or alcohol drinks by Fruit Infused Water, and add the healthy beverages in your routine every day. And remember that

Healthy Mind+ Healthy Lifestyle= Happy Life.

Everything You Need to Know About Detox Drinks

* * *

First of all, I want to tell you the importance of detox in your life. Not only is detox drinks for weight loss, but also is it essential for your daily life.

Why do we need detox drink/tea?

Nowadays, the environment is polluted, the food is dirty. Thus, we unintentionally absorbed toxic or pollutant into our body. This is the reason which causes many diseases about liver, kidneys, lungs, etc. Drinking detox tea will help us raise body resistance to avoid these diseases as well as help our body released the pollutants that we take in from the outside factors. Moreover, if you are on the diet, it's really good for you to drop your weight by boosting the metabolism and burning fat storage. It not only help you release pollutants, lose your weight but also make you become beautiful with a nice skin because it provides essential vitamins, and minerals for your body.

A fresh, clean and healthy body!

When do we drink detox tea?

We will use detox drinks for weight loss in the middle of meals to reduce hungry feeling and craving.

3 Detox tea benefits

Detox herbal tea/drink will make you become healthier and

fresheSr without using coffee. What do you think if you will replace your favorite drink (coffee) to a natural tea, which does not cause side effects as coffee? It's really awesome, right?

Remove the body toxins & Boost the immune system

As I mentioned before, currently, there are many outside pollutants absorbed into your body, such as the pollution, food toxic, etc... And the subjective factors are your bad daily habits. You often drink wine, alcohol, caffeine, or preservatives? That's not good for your health! You are taking a lot of toxins in your body that can make you become weaker step by step. Even it will be dangerous for your life if you abuse them. Let you give up your bad habits and drink detox tea regularly because detox herbal tea will help you release the pollutants you absorbed out of your body.

The immune system is one of the most important roles of our body. It helps us become healthier and protects us against viruses and bacteria. Detox tea is naturally high in antioxidants which get rid you of free radicals that can decrease the effectiveness of your immune system. Detox herbal tea maximizes your body's defense.

Prevent your craving & Increase your metabolism

Have you realized some have a bigger craving than others? And sometimes your craving changes also for low to high or the other way round? What does this mean? It is important these days when eating more protein and fibre as these are beginning to drop in many diets. In place we are eating a lot more carbohydrates and this is becoming increasingly more and more popular. Often these are also simple sugars, which are even more of an issue.

The right types of foods give you vitality throughout the day and you are better able to maintain your energy rather than short bursts which often lead you to be eating even more of the wrong foods. Natural detox tea suppresses the appetite in various ways this way you have less and less cravings. If you also increase protein, fiber and low carb vegetables you are definitely on track. The tea also raises your metabolism so that you are better able to burn more calories and your metabolism is not going through sleepy periods. The perfect blend also decreases fat storage in the body.

Improves Your Digestion

We all know that digestion is essential and important for our wellbeing. Detox herbal tea assists in digestion and improves our body's ability to effectively digest and break down our food and eventually lead to keeping what we need and eliminating all the waste form the body. Sometimes we feel bloated and uncomfortable and an improved digestion can be a welcome relief, which can also sometimes lead to constipation.

As we want to maximize the digestion efficiency, we need to take herbal tea in the morning and in the evening, about half an hour before breakfast and dinner. As well as improving digestion, it is the right time to suppress your appetite also, we all know how we can go overboard so easily, way past the moment we are no longer hungry, even past full.

So if you have been wondering how to lose weight fast or the best way to lose weight and slim fast, then buy a packet of our amazing liquid diet, a true detox drink and begin to lose weight in a week. Detox tea really does work and benefits you in many great ways, including losing weight as well as leaving you feel great and energized.

The most common reason people choose to try detox tea is the decision to start a new and healthy routine – and an organic tea detox or 'Teatox' is a smart place to begin. Drinking an organic detox tea has a number of beneficial effects that will help you to instantly feel more energized vibrant and less bloated.

Note, using detox tea combine with diet and workout plan to get the best result.

Remember that: **Diet plan + Workout schedule + Natural supplement = Perfect Body!**

Health & Benefits of Ingredients

* * *

Strawberries

Berries are packed with antioxidants that fight cancer, lower the risk of diabetes, boost brain function, and help regulate and lower bad cholesterol and blood pressure. Berries are also rich in pectin, a form of soluble fiber that can lower total cholesterol levels. Strawberries and raspberries are also a good source of folate, a nutrient needed by expectant mothers to stave off birth defects. Fiber in berries relieves constipation and the anthocyanins in berries repair aging skin.

Pineapple

Pineapple contains an enzyme called bromelain that aids in digestion and cleans the blood while also helping in the breakdown of protein. Pineapple is also anti-inflammatory, so this juice is particularly great for those with arthritis or joint pain. Pineapple also contains manganese, which serves to regulate blood glucose and boost your immune system alongside the plentiful amounts of Vitamin C.

Apples

The phytonutrients in apples help to regulate blood sugar by breaking down complex carbohydrates into simple sugars that are easy for your body to digest. Apples help with elimination and weight loss due to a high level of pectin, which is a type of soluble fiber. Pectin lowers blood fat, making apples a heart-healthy addition to any juice.

Watermelon

Watermelon is an ideal food when cleansing. It makes a rejuvenating blood tonic, as it is very alkalizing, antibacterial, antioxidant, anticoagulation, and serves as a diuretic, laxative, and digestive aid. Watermelon is also a good source of beta-carotene, vitamin C, and potassium. It has half the sugar of an apple, but tastes sweeter, as it is over 90% water! Watermelon has been known to alleviate depression and helps with hangovers, mouth sores, sore throat, and urethral pain, too!

Cucumber

Cucumbers have amazing anti-inflammatory qualities that can reduce swelling, as well assoothe and soften skin tissue. They are also an excellent source of silica, a trace mineral that strengthens the skin's connective tissue. Cucumbers will alkalize, cleanse the skin, and release toxins from the body, all while providing the body with hydration, as cucumbers are mostly water! Silica in cucumbers will keep your hair and nails strong, refresh and heal the gums and mouth, and lower uric acid levels in the body, which will keep your kidneys in shape. Cucumbers are also packed with vitamins A, B, and C, which will make you feel radiant and energetic while protecting your immune system. Magnesium, potassium, and silicone all combine to heal and refresh the skin, your largest organ, as well as your body!

Lemon

Lemon is a bright and refreshing flavor that always leaves us with more mental clarity, but there are many physical benefits as well! Lemon can clear up acne when ingested or applied topically, and also relieve canker sores with proven antibacterial and anti-fungal agents. Any time you're feeling a cold coming on, sip on some immune-boosting lemon water with honey to keep it at bay!

Lime

Limes are high in calcium and folate, and inhibit melanin production, which will leave you with younger, healthier skin! They are also anti-carcinogenic, protecting you from cancer as well as kidney stones! Swap your lemon for a lime every now and again; they're worth it!

Basil

Basil is anti-inflammatory AND antibacterial! It fights against free radicals and protects the heart with a generous dose of magnesium, so don't hesitate to get a whole plant of it and eat it as fresh as possible.

Mint

Mint aids with digestion, nausea, headaches, respiratory disorders, coughs, asthma, depression, fatigue, and acne, as well as giving you some pretty amazing breath! Mint tea or water infused with mint should definitely become a routine!

Ginger

Ginger does wonder for digestion and will detoxify your gastrointestinal tract in a variety of ways. For one, ginger improves nutrient absorption by stimulating gastric and pancreatic enzyme secretion and relieves stomachaches, pain, and inflammation. Ginger is powerful: regular consumption of ginger slows the growth of colorectal cancer cells!

Cinnamon

Cinnamon regulates blood sugar and improves blood glucose

control. Just half a teaspoon of cinnamon every day can significantly reduce blood sugar levels, triglycerides, bad cholesterol, and total cholesterol levels in diabetics. Cinnamon also improves digestion, relieves congestion, and can reduce inflammation, including relieving pain and stiffness in joints due to arthritis.

Apple Cider Vinegar

Apple cider vinegar is rich in acetic acid, which regulates blood sugar levels by slowing the digestion of starch. It is also rich in ash, which regulates the body's pH levels (especially great if you're a caffeine or alcohol drinker!). It also helps to clear up skin!

One: Detox Water

* * *

Herbal - Based Recipes
***

Beetroot Curry Leaves Detox Drink

A healthy, detox drink with beetroot, curry leaves, lemon and ginger.
*Servings: 8 | **Prep**: 10 m | **Cook**: 6 h | **Ready In**: 6 h 10 m*

Ingredients
- ✓ Beetroot- 1 (peeled and sliced)
- ✓ Curry leaves - ½ cup
- ✓ Lemon - 1 (thinly sliced)
- ✓ Ginger - 2 tablespoon (grated)
- ✓ Water - 8 glasses

Directions
1. Boil 2 glasses of water with curry leaves in it. Let it cool down completely.
2. Now add this curry leaves water along with sliced beetroots, lemon, ginger and remaining glasses of water in a glass jar. Mix it well.
3. Close the jar and leave it overnight or for minimum 6 hours.
4. Strain the infused water and enjoy.

Notes
- ✓ Refrigerate if you stay in a warm place.

Belly Slimming Detox Water

Get rid of that midsection in a jiffy by chugging down the best detox water ever put in a jar. By relying steadfastly on this brew, a tight little waist is just around the corner.

Ingredients

- ✓ Ice
- ✓ Water
- ✓ 3 Basil leaves roughly chopped
- ✓ 1 strawberry sliced
- ✓ 3 - 5 slices of cucumber

Directions

1. Combine all the ingredients in a large glass
2. Let it sit for 5 minutes at least
3. Enjoy

Berry Rosemary

Servings: 6 | Prep: 60 m | Ready In: 1 h

Ingredients

- ✓ 1 cup mixed fresh or frozen berries (strawberries, raspberries, blackberries, blueberries)
- ✓ 1 sprig fresh rosemary

Directions

1. Place in a carafe, jar, or pitcher and fill with water. Refrigerate until ready to drink, at least an hour to allow flavor to infuse the water.
2. Keeps for 1-2 days in the fridge. Can be refilled with water two or three times, or until flavor dissipates.

Blueberry Lavender Water

Here we go! This one is a special elixir that cures the mind and body alike. The blueberries naturally expel unwanted toxins in droves, and they release ample B vitamins into the system, which promotes energetic exercise alongside active engagement.

Servings*: 8*

Ingredients

- ✓ 1/2 pint Blueberries
- ✓ Edible Flowers (use Lavender Flowers) - to taste
- ✓ 64 ounces Water

Directions

1. Add Fruits and edible flowers to a pitcher of water.
2. Cover, and chill for at least 30 minutes.
3. Strain, then add ice and pour into tall glasses and serve.

Citrus and Mint Infused Water

When mommy wants to look her finest, she turns to a diet that consists solely of this mega mint detox water. Her kids will also learn to love the lively drink.

Servings*: 4 | **Prep***: 5 m | ***Ready In***: 5 m

Ingredients

- ✓ 1 large Orange
- ✓ 2 large Lemons
- ✓ 2 quarts Water
- ✓ 10 Mint Leaves

Directions

1. Wash and slice lemons and oranges into thin rings. Break the mint leaves into small pieces. Place ingredients into a jar.

2. Fill the jar with ice and water, let the water soak up the flavor of citrus and mint for at least 10 minutes. Btw, my kids love this infused water.

Clementine Cinnamon Cilantro Detox Drink

A refreshing way to keep you healthy and hydrated!
Servings: 8 | Prep: 10 m | Cook: 6 h | Ready In: 6 h 10 m

Ingredients
- ✓ Clementine - 1 (thinly sliced)
- ✓ Cinnamon - ½ stick (break it into few pieces)
- ✓ Cilantro/Coriander leaves - ½ cup
- ✓ Water - 8 glasses

Directions
1. Add all ingredients in a glass jar and mix well.
2. Close the jar and refrigerate it overnight or for minimum 6 hours.
3. Strain the infused water and enjoy.

Cucumber Lemon Lime Basil Infused Water

Ingredients
- ✓ 32 oz. canning jar
- ✓ 1 medium cucumber, cut into slices
- ✓ 1 medium lemon, sliced
- ✓ 1 medium lime sliced
- ✓ ½ cup of fresh basil

Directions
1. Add the cucumber, sliced fruit and basil to the canning jar.

2. Mash them down a bit to get the juice out of them. The more juice, the more flavor in your water!
3. Fill the jar with water and let it refrigerate overnight.
4. Enjoy ice cold!

Cucumber Lemon Mint Ginger Detox Drink

A healthy, detox drink with cucumber, lemon, ginger and mint.
***Servings:** 8 | **Prep:** 10 m | **Cook:** 6 h | **Ready In:** 6 h 10 m*

Ingredients
- ✓ Cucumber - 1 (thinly sliced)
- ✓ Lemon - 2 (thinly sliced)
- ✓ Ginger - 2 tablespoon (grated)
- ✓ Mint leaves - ½ cup
- ✓ Water - 8 glasses

Directions
1. Add all ingredients in a glass jar and mix well.
2. Close the jar and leave it overnight or for minimum 6 hours.
3. Strain the infused water and enjoy.

Cucumber Melon Mint

***Servings:** 6 | **Prep:** 60 m | **Ready In:** 1 h*

Ingredients
- ✓ ¼ to ½ large cucumber
- ✓ 2 slices cantaloupe
- ✓ 1 handful fresh mint
- ✓ 1-2 quarts water

Directions

1. Place in a carafe, jar, or pitcher and fill with water. Refrigerate until ready to drink, at least an hour to allow flavor to infuse the water.
2. Keeps for 2-3 days in the fridge. Can be refilled with water two or three times, or until flavor dissipates.

Cucumber, Lemon & Mint Water

Cucumber, lemon, and mint detox water helps flush out of your body. The lemon and mint both aid in digestion, and the cucumber re-hydrates along with having anti-inflammatory properties.

Ingredients

- ✓ 2L water
- ✓ 1 medium cucumber
- ✓ 1 lemon
- ✓ 10+ mint leaves
- ✓ (optional) 2 inch piece of ginger for some extra zest + digestive benefits
- ✓ (optional) 5+ strawberries for some added flavor, and your water will turn pink!

Directions

- ✓ Wash veggies. Slice cucumber & lemon, add mint leaves, peeled ginger & sliced strawberries if desired. Let steep in fridge for a minimum of 1 hr. For best results leave overnight. Detoxing made easy, Enjoy!

Fat Flush Detox Drink

With the girl that is always on the go, there is no better friend than a green tea beverage. For thousands of years, Chinese cultures have used this ancient plant to lose weight and gain energy. It delivers an awakening jolt with its natural caffeine reserves, and the ability to do more fitness activities makes shedding weight a double pronged effort.

Ingredients
- ✓ Water
- ✓ 1 Lime
- ✓ 1 Green Tea Bag
- ✓ ¼ Cup of Mint Leaves

Directions
1. Fill a large mason jar (about 24 oz of water) - add tea bag (I do a cold brew)
2. Allow to sit in the fridge for 30 minutes
3. Cut up lime and chop up mint
4. Place in the water
5. Cover and take out tea bag
6. Place in the fridge for 30 more minutes
7. Enjoy!

Flavored Strawberry Fruit Water

Treat your taste buds to a fruit-filled rainbow. Cavalcades of sweet natural treats are infused in this energetic ensemble.

Ingredients
- ✓ 1 each of the following fruits: apple, lemon, orange, pear
- ✓ 4 large strawberries
- ✓ Handful of raspberries
- ✓ Handful of mint leaves
- ✓ 1 half-gallon of water

Directions

- ✓ Cut large slices or thin wedges of each fruit; place them in a large glass pitcher and add cold water. Refrigerate 2 hours and serve over ice in tall glasses.

Fruit Infused Water

Fruit infused waters are a great alternative to water because they taste amazing and they're made with super healthy ingredients.
Prep: *5 m* | **Ready In**: *5 m*

Ingredients

- ✓ 1 sliced orange
- ✓ 6 sliced strawberries
- ✓ 10 mint leaves
- ✓ 4 cups water (1 l)

Directions

- ✓ Place the sliced fruits and the mint leaves in a glass jar, pour the water and refrigerate for at least 1 or 2 hours (can even do overnight). The longer it sits, the more flavorful the water will be.

Lavender Vanilla Lemonade

Soothe your mind and body with this amazing lavender vanilla lemonade. Perfect for those DIY at-home spa days.

Ingredients

- ✓ 2 cups filtered water
- ✓ 1 cup vanilla sugar (I sometimes substitute stevia here for a sugar free option, you'll have to adjust stevia to taste. It won't be 1 cup)

✓ 1 tablespoon dried lavender

✓ 1 tablespoon homemade vanilla bean extract

✓ 2/3 cup fresh organic lemon juice (about 3-4 lemons depending on size)

✓ 6 cups filtered water

Directions

1. Cut and juice 3 to 4 lemons or until you get about 2/3 cup fresh juice. Pour into a pitcher that holds two quarts liquid.

2. In a small pot add 2 cups filtered water, sugar, lavender, and vanilla extract. Bring to a simmer stirring occasionally. When comes to simmer immediately turn off heat. Remove from heat. Let steep 5-10 minutes.

3. When the mixture has cooled slightly, strain vanilla, sugar, lavender liquid into pitcher with lemon juice.

4. Finally pour remaining filtered water into pitcher, stir and taste. We like our lemonade more tart and sweet. We fill our cups to the top with ice so when the ice melts the lemonade is diluted just perfectly. Garnish with a lemon slice and lavender sprig and serve chilled! I love how the steeped lavender turns the lemonade the slightest hue of pink. This is just so refreshing!

Lemon and Mint Detox Water

Lemon water detox methods have reached a zenith with this thirst-quenching diet recipe. For those that love sugary drinks, this tasty blend can permanently replace sodas and fruit juices.

Ingredients

✓ 6 cups water

✓ 2 lemons, thinly sliced

✓ sprigs of mint

✓ ice

Directions

1. Combine all ingredients in a pitcher and put in the fridge for two hours to allow the water to infuse.
2. You can also squeeze in the juice of one lemon to intensify flavor a bit.
3. Serve cold.

Mango Mint Infused Water

Ingredients

✓ ½ mango, peeled and sliced

✓ 1 handful fresh basil, washed well

✓ 1-2 quarts water

Directions

1. Place in a carafe, jar, or pitcher and fill with water. Refrigerate until ready to drink, at least an hour to allow flavor to infuse the water.
2. Keeps for 2-3 days in the fridge. Can be refilled with water two or three times, or until flavor dissipates.

Mexican Mojito

Servings: 1 | Cook: 5 m | Ready In: 5 m

Ingredients

✓ 3 sprigs of mint

✓ 1/2 lime, cut into three wedges

✓ 2-3 teaspoons sugar, depending on how sweet you like your drink

✓ 1 1/2 ounces white tequila

- ✓ handful of ice
- ✓ 1/2 cup sparkling water or seltzer water
- ✓ slice lime and mint leaves for garnish (optional)

Directions

- ✓ In a glass, muddle the mint, lime wedges and sugar (I use a wooden spoon). Add the tequila and stir to mix and dissolve the sugar. Add ice and then the sparkling water. Garnish with a slice of lime and mint leaves, if desired.

Naturally Flavored Fruit & Herb Detox Water

Ladies, get ready to give up carbonated sodas once and for all! This deliciously detoxifying potion is the world's top substitute for mass-produced bottled beverages.

Servings*: 6-8*

Ingredients

- ✓ Fruit - 2 cups berries, citrus, melons, pineapple...most fruits will work (see recommended amounts in Directions)
- ✓ Herbs - a sprig of mint, basil, sage, rosemary, tarragon, thyme, or lavender
- ✓ Water (tap or filtered)
- ✓ Ice

Directions

Supplies needed:

- ✓ 2 quart pitcher or jar with lid; muddler or wooden spoon

General formula for whatever fruit/herb combo you desire.

1. If using herbs, add a sprig of fresh herbs to jar/pitcher; press and twist with muddler or handle of wooden spoon to bruise leaves and release flavor; don't pulverize the herbs into bits.

2. Add approx. 2 cups of fruit to jar/pitcher; press and twist with muddler or handle of wooden spoon, just enough to release some of the juices
3. Fill jar/pitcher with ice cubes.
4. Add water to top of jar/pitcher.
5. Cover and refrigerate for up to 3 days.

Suggested flavor combinations:

1. ALL CITRUS (no herbs) -- Slice 1 orange, 1 lime, 1 lemon into rounds, then cut the rounds in half. Add to jar and proceed with muddling, add ice & water.
2. RASPBERRY LIME (no herbs) -- Quarter 2 limes; with your hands, squeeze the juice into the jar, then throw in the squeezed lime quarters. Add 2 cups raspberries. Muddle, add ice & water.
3. PINEAPPLE MINT -- Add a sprig of mint to the jar (you can throw in the whole sprig; or, remove the leaves from the sprig, if you prefer to have the mint swimming around and distributing in the jar). Muddle the mint. Add 2 cups pineapple pieces, muddle, add ice & water.
4. BLACKBERRY SAGE -- Add sage sprig to jar and muddle. Add 2 cups blackberries; muddle, add ice & water.
5. WATERMELON ROSEMARY -- Add rosemary sprig to jar & muddle. Add 2 cups watermelon cubes; muddle, add ice and water.

New Year Detox Water

Ok, so it's not even close to the New Year so you can just call this one the New You Detox Water.

Ingredients
✓ 1 Large Pitcher of Spring Water

- ✓ Raspberries
- ✓ Peeled Grapefruit
- ✓ Sliced Cucumbers
- ✓ Sliced Pears
- ✓ Fresh Mint
- ✓ *additional add-ins
- ✓ Sliced Lemons
- ✓ Sliced Limes
- ✓ Cranberries
- ✓ Blueberries

Directions

1. Combine ingredients into pitcher. Allow to chill in refrigerator for 1-2 hours. Drink throughout the day.
2. Make a new pitcher each day.

Peach Mint Water

This curbs your appetite and helps fill up your tummy to avoid mindless snacking, naturally. Mint is cooling and helps suppress your appetite. You can enhance the flavor by adding a bit of vanilla.

Ingredients

- ✓ 1 sprig of Mint or you can muddle a few mint leaves
- ✓ 12-14 peach slices, frozen
- ✓ Water

Directions

- ✓ Muddle a few mint leaves (crush it coarsely in mortar and pestle). Add peaches and now top it up with water. You can garnish with peaches and mint leaves. This is one of the best mint infused water recipes to try out.

Raspberry and Mint Scented Water

Servings: 6

Ingredients

- ✓ 2 litres cold spring water, or filtered tap water
- ✓ 2 Tablespoons raspberries, fresh or frozen
- ✓ 2 tablespoons fresh mint leaves
- ✓ 1 lime

Directions

1. To get more flavour and juice out of your lime, microwave for 30 seconds. When cool, slice
2. Place raspberries, mint, lime and water in a large jug. Stir and serve!

Refreshing Citrus and Cucumber Detox Water

This enriching brew will fuel your core with hefty doses of vitamin C. This health positive compound purifies the entire digestive system while also flushing out toxins from the liver.
***Servings:** 10 | **Prep:** 10 m | **Ready In:** 10 m*

Ingredients

- ✓ 2-3 liters water
- ✓ 2 large oranges, sliced
- ✓ 1 lemon, sliced
- ✓ ½ large cucumber, sliced
- ✓ 1 handful of fresh mint

Directions

1. Put oranges, lemon and cucumber in the water pitcher. Using a long spoon, gently mash fruits/veggies; this will release more flavor.

2. Take the mint, and gently mash it to release the natural oils; add to the pitcher.
3. Add water to the pitcher, and stir to begin the infusion process.
4. Drink/serve immediately, or store in the refrigerator for up to 2 days.

Notes

✓ This water also tastes great when infused overnight; if doing so, consider removing the rinds from the lemon and oranges. This will cut down on the bitterness.

Refreshing Detox Drink

For those that resist tradition detox methods, watermelon water may be the cure. It is filled with antioxidants, and the fluids have been shown to expunge unwanted toxins. Melons make detoxifying accessible to all demographics.

Ingredients

✓ 1/2 Cup Watermelon Cut into chunks
✓ 4-5 Mint leaves
✓ 1/2 lemon cut into slices

Directions

1. Fill a glass with ice and cold water (cold water helps speed metabolism and tastes great)
2. Add watermelon, mint and melon to water
3. Let sit for 20 - 30 minutes then drink
4. Enjoy!

Rose Mint Water

Ingredients

- ✓ 4 mint sprigs, plus more for garnish
- ✓ 1/2 teaspoons rose water (available in the drink section at many grocery stores)
- ✓ 2 quarts water

Directions

1. Add mint sprigs and rose water to a jar or bottle.
2. Add water and rose water; cover and chill until ready to serve.

Rosemary Grapefruit Water

Do you want to flush out your system after an overindulgence and immediately get your mind and body back on the healthy track? Well then look no further! As you probably know, living in the very social New York City, our clients at times come to us after a night or weekend of social engagements and want to minimize the damage from the overindulgences, so we're armed and ready to help! ;) Not only is this ingredient combo the perfect pair for a refreshing and thirst quenching drink, but it will also help to flush bloat and toxins.

Servings: 2

Ingredients

- ✓ 32 oz water
- ✓ 1 grapefruit
- ✓ 1 sprig of fresh rosemary

Directions

1. Cut the rind away from the grapefruit (leave a little rind for added flavor) and cut the fruit into slices.
2. Fill a jar or infuser bottle with water, then lower the fruit into the water (instead of pouring water over the fruit).
3. Infuse for 2 hours at room temperature and up to 24 hours in your refrigerator.

Skinny Detox Water Recipe

Ingredients

- ✓ Lemon (Lemons are natural energizers plus it kick starts that metabolism)
- ✓ Lime (natural energizers helps your metabolism)
- ✓ Grapefruit - (natural energizers with a bit of sweetness)
- ✓ Cucumber (Helps give the drink an extremely refreshing taste (it is pretty addicting))
- ✓ Fresh Mint (Helps your breath and helps you tummy work better)
- ✓ Ice
- ✓ Water

Directions

1. In a glass – combine water and ice (about ¾th of the glass)
2. Add lemon, lime, grapefruit, cucumber and mint till the drink is full
3. For my mason jar I used 2 full slices of lemon, 1 slice of grapefruit, 2 small slices of lime ,3 slices of cucumber and 6 mint leaves
4. Stir and left sit for 5 minutes (keep the ingredients in the drink while you enjoy it)

Slim Down Detox Water

This great detox water not only rids your body of toxins but helps to flush fat from your body as well.
Servings: 1-8 oz glass | Prep: 10 m

Ingredients

- ✓ ½ gallon spring water
- ✓ ½ grapefruit, sliced
- ✓ ½ cucumber, sliced
- ✓ 2-3 mint leaves
- ✓ ½ lemon, sliced
- ✓ ½ lime, sliced

Directions

1. Combine all ingredients in a pitcher.
2. Allow the ingredients to chill in the refrigerator for 1-2 hours before serving. Drink throughout the day or discard after 24 hours.

Nutrition Information

- ✓ Calories: 7
- ✓ Fat: 0g
- ✓ Carbohydrates: 1g
- ✓ Fiber: 1g
- ✓ Protein: 0g
- ✓ Sugars: 0g
- ✓ Sodium: 0mg
- ✓ Vitamin A: 1%
- ✓ Vitamin C: 11%
- ✓ Calcium: 0%
- ✓ Iron: 0%
- ✓ WWP+: 0 points

Springtime Strawberry Spa Water

If you want a drink that mimics the fancy beverages served in health spas, try this homemade detox water.

Ingredients

- ✓ 1 gallon of water
- ✓ 1 large lemon thinly sliced
- ✓ 1 small cucumber, thinly sliced
- ✓ 6 medium sized strawberries, hulled and thinly sliced
- ✓ 3 small sprigs of fresh herbs - basil or mint is nice

Directions

1. Place all the sliced fruits and veggies into a pitcher.
2. Add the sprigs of herbs, and fill the pitcher with water.
3. The water tastes best after 6-8 hours in the refrigerator, but it will keep up to 2 days in the fridge.

Notes

- ✓ You can add as much fresh herbs as you'd like. This infused water is also delicious without any fresh herbs if you don't have any handy!

Strawberry Basil Lemonade

Servings: 10-12 | Prep: 15 m | Ready In: 15 m

Ingredients

- ✓ 1 can of Minute Maid Pink Lemonade or your favorite lemonade
- ✓ 1 lb of strawberries
- ✓ 1 lemon, sliced
- ✓ 1 small handful of basil, optional
- ✓ Ice as needed

Directions

1. Prepare Minute Maid Lemonade according to instructions on the can - 1 can of concentrate and 4⅓ cans of water, stirred together.

2. Wash 1 lb of strawberries. Remove stems and cut them in half.
3. Blend strawberries in a blender or food processor. Finely chop basil and add it to the mix.
4. Stir strawberry mixture and lemon slices into the lemonade. Add lots of ice and enjoy!

Strawberry Flavored Water

Say good riddance to the summers filled with unhealthy lemonade. Kiss the bellyaches goodbye by switching to the joy of this stunningly sweet strawberry detox water. A rich lemon core purifies the entire digestive arena, and it masks most of the complex flavor with a brilliant spectacle of sour.

Prep: 5 m | Ready In: 5 m

Ingredients

- 4-6 strawberries, hulled and quartered
- ½ lemon, sliced
- Small handful of basil, scrunched
- Ice and cold filtered water

Directions

1. Fill your juice pitcher to the top with ice and fruit.
2. Slightly scrunch up the basil so it releases it's flavor. Cover with cold filtered water.
3. This water is best if you let the water infuse at least 1 hour. If you're inpatient (like me), poke a few holes in your fruit with a fork for instant flavor.

Strawberry Infused Vitamin Water

This hydrating and antioxidant infused-water boasts flavor and skin enhancing nutrients, not to mention a beautiful presentation! Enjoy this refreshing and seasonal anti-inflammatory drink!

Ingredients
- ✓ 1 cup strawberries
- ✓ 2 cups watermelon, cubed
- ✓ 2 sprigs fresh rosemary
- ✓ dash of course salt
- ✓ filtered water

Directions
1. Muddle the strawberries and rosemary in a bowl.
2. Add the muddled ingredients and the watermelon to a large pitcher. Pour water over the ingredients and stir.
3. Refrigerate for 4-6 hours, and enjoy!

Strawberry, Lime, Cucumber and Mint Water

Jazz up your daily hydration with this infused water. Strawberries add a little sweetness, while cucumber, mint, and lime make the water taste so refreshing and bright!

*Serving size: ½ gallon | **Cook:** 10 m | **Ready In:** 10 m*

Ingredients
- ✓ 1 cup sliced strawberries
- ✓ 1 cup sliced cucumbers
- ✓ 2 limes, sliced
- ✓ ¼ cup fresh mint leaves
- ✓ Ice cubes

✓ Water

Directions

✓ In a half-gallon jar, or a 2 quart pitcher, layer the strawberries, cucumbers, lime slices, and mint leaves with the ice cubes. Fill jar or pitcher with water. Let chill for 10 minutes, and then enjoy!

Notes

✓ I can get 2-4 fill-ups out of one batch of flavorings, but you might want to change out your flavorings sooner for stronger flavor.
✓ Feel free to use sparkling water instead of still water.
✓ Obviously, the longer the water sits, the stronger the flavor. It's mild at first, but after a few hours (or overnight) it's quite strong.

Strawberry-Basil Infused Water

Servings: 10

Ingredients

✓ 2 cups of water or sparkling water
✓ 2 cups of ice
✓ 1 cup strawberries, sliced
✓ handful basil

Directions

✓ Combine all in a large mason jar or jug and drink immediately or let sit in fridge for 1-4 hours to soak in additional flavor.

Stress Relieving Detox Water

Ingredients

- ✓ 5 strawberries
- ✓ 1/2 cup pineapple
- ✓ 1 to 2 teaspoons apple cider vinegar*
- ✓ 4 to 5 medium basil leaves
- ✓ 1/2 cup ice

Directions

1. Drop (ingredients) in the bottom of the pitcher, cover with ice about 1/2 way up then add filtered water and stir. Place the detox water in the fridge for a few hours before drinking (2-4 glasses per day!).

2. Ingredients listed are for a large 2 quart pitcher, reduce by half to use a 22-32 oz bell/mason jar.

3. All done! Enjoy!!

Watermelon and Mint Detox Water

This enriching brew will fuel your core with hefty doses of vitamin C. This health positive compound purifies the entire digestive system while also flushing out toxins from the liver.

Prep: *10 m*

Ingredients

- ✓ Raspberry (or strawberry) lemon - any berry paired with lemon ends up with a light lemonade flavor!
- ✓ Watermelon mint - super refreshing!
- ✓ Tropical (mango pineapple) - this one comes out sweeter than the others, but in a totally good way!
- ✓ Citrus cucumber (lemon, lime, orange, cucumber)
- ✓ Other fruits to try: apples, honeydew, cantalope, blueberries, blackberries, peaches
- ✓ Try fresh herbs too! Rosemary, basil, mint

Directions

✓ Add desired fruits to a pitcher and then fill with water. Allow fruit to soak for 2-8 hours in the fridge and then enjoy! You can add as much or as little fruit as you'd prefer. Add more fruit for more flavor and sweetness for your waters.

Watermelon Rosemary Water

Ingredients

✓ 2 cups cubed watermelon
✓ 1 sprig rosemary
✓ 2 quarts water

Directions

1. Put rosemary in a jar and massage gently with a wooden spoon.
2. Add watermelon to jar and gently mash some of the cubes with a wooden spoon.
3. Pour in water, cover, and chill until ready to serve.

Weight Loss Detox Drink

This is a signature recipe for aficionados of the weight loss game. If the situation is urgent, desperate measures may be needed. Luckily, the garden may hold the clues to a successful slimming venture.

Ingredients

✓ 2 quarts water
✓ 1 Lemon
✓ 1 Cucumber
✓ 1 Tablespoon grated Fresh Ginger
✓ 1 Lime

✓ Fresh Mint (about 10-15 leaves)

Directions

1. Cut the lemon, lime and cucumber into thin slices with peels
2. Grate the ginger
3. Combine all of the ingredients and stir
4. Place the detox water in the fridge for a few hours and drink 2-3 glasses a day!

Fruit - Based Recipes
* * *

Blackberry Peach Detox Water

Ingredients & Directions

This recipe is a bit more complicated than just adding some fruit to water. You need to make simple syrup from ¾ cup of sugar and 2 cups of water. Once that's done, mix in ½ cup of blackberries and 2 peaches, sliced. You can also add a couple of cups of peach orchard juice to give it more of a peachy flavor. The blackberries in this have wonderful antioxidant properties and peaches are great for helping to cleanse your systems from your colon to your digestive tract. Keep this in the fridge and enjoy it all day.

Blueberry and Raspberry Infused Water

Ingredients
- ✓ One 8 oz. canning jar
- ✓ 1/4 cup of fresh blueberries, left whole
- ✓ 1/4 cup of fresh raspberries, left whole

Directions
1. Add the fresh blueberries and raspberries to your canning jar. Next, gently mash the fruit down with a fork or a spoon so the juice leaks out and infuses your water. If you own a muddler, that would work great too.
2. Once the fruit is mashed, fill the jar with water, place the cover on, shake it once or twice and place in the fridge

overnight. The longer you let it set, the better that water will taste.

Blueberry Orange Water

Ingredients
- ✓ 6 cups water
- ✓ 2 mandarin oranges, cut into wedges
- ✓ a handful of blueberries
- ✓ ice

Directions
1. Combine all ingredients in a pitcher and put in the fridge for 2-24 hours to allow the water to infuse.
2. You can also squeeze in the juice of one mandarin orange and muddle the blueberries to intensify flavor a bit.
3. Serve cold.

Blueberry-Lime Infused Water

Ingredients
- ✓ 2 cups of water or sparkling water
- ✓ 2 cups of ice
- ✓ 1 cup blueberries, whole
- ✓ 1 1/2 limes, sliced

Directions
- ✓ Combine all in a large mason jar or jug and drink immediately or let sit in fridge for 1-4 hours to soak in additional flavor.

Charcoal Black Lemonade

Prep: 10 m | Ready In: 10 m

Ingredients

- ✓ 4 cups filtered water
- ✓ ¼ cup freshly squeezed lemon juice (more or less to taste)
- ✓ Stevia to taste (I used about 15 drops)
- ✓ ¼ teaspoon (about 1 capsule) activated charcoal

Directions

- ✓ Whisk together all of the ingredients until desired taste is achieved. Serve over ice.

Chia Fruit Water

Make your own natural energy drink with water, fruit and chia seeds!
Prep: *1 m* | **Ready In**: *1 m*

Ingredients

- ✓ a large bottle or jar
- ✓ cold water
- ✓ fruit of your choice (I used strawberries, lemon and lime)
- ✓ 1 tablespoon chia seeds

Directions

1. Add all the ingredients to the bottle or jar and shake well.
2. Refrigerate for 10 minutes and shake again.
3. Drink within a couple of hours.

Cinnamon Apple Water

Ingredients

- ✓ 1 Thinly sliced apple
- ✓ 1 Cinnamon Stick if you like

Directions

- ✓ Put the apple slices in a big jug, and top it up with water and ice.

Cranberry Orange Detox Water

Drink your nutrients in this simple to make, delicious cranberry orange detox water. Lemon aids in digestion, while cranberries exhibit incredible anti-inflammatory properties.

Prep: 5 m | Cook: 5 m | Ready In: 20 m

Ingredients

- ✓ 1 Blood Orange, cut into slices
- ✓ 1 Lemon, cut into slices
- ✓ Handful of Fresh Cranberries
- ✓ 2 Liters Water

Directions

1. Cut orange and lemon into slices.
2. Put orange, lemon, and cranberries into a pitcher and add about two liters of water. Let fruit "steep" for about 15-20 minutes.
3. Serve in glasses with fruit, if desired.
4. Enjoy!

Notes

- ✓ If there aren't any blood oranges to be found, use cara cara or navel oranges instead.
- ✓ Steep detox water overnight for maximum benefits.

Day Spa Apple Cinnamon Detox Water

Makes one big pitcher, re-fill water 3-4 times before replacing apples and cinnamon

Ingredients
- ✓ 1 Apple thinly slice (Whatever your favorite is)
- ✓ 1 Cinnamon Stick

Directions
- ✓ Drop apple slices in the bottom of the pitcher (save a few to drop in your glass later) and then the cinnamon stick, cover with ice about 1/2 way through then with water. Place in the fridge for 10 minutes before serving.

My Notes
- ✓ I found that with my pitcher I add 2 apples and 2 cinnamon sticks. I really like the cinnamon taste so I keep a stick in my large cup and just keep refilling and leave it in there. I have had some suggestions to boil the cinnamon and/or apple to help release some of the juices. I haven't tried this yet but I plan to and will comment here when I can. I have tried different apples and my found that Fuji which was recommended is my favorite. We had some Granny Smith in the house and it didn't give the same taste I like. I don't eat the apples just keep refilling 3 or 4 times to get the taste. I drink this all day long instead of my coffee that I use to drink or flavored waters. I'm still eating a healthy diet and exercising. I'm just using this as a boost and to help me with my weight loss goal).

Day Spa Mango Ginger Water

Makes 4 liters of Mango Ginger Detox Water, refill 4 liter pitcher 2-4 times until flavor is lost.

Ingredients

- ✓ 1 inch Ginger Root, peeled and sliced
- ✓ 1 cup Frozen Mango- fresh is fine too

Directions

1. To peel the ginger use the back of a spoon or a vegetable peeler, just peel the part that you will be using.
2. Using a sharp knife slice ginger into 3-4 coin sized slices.
3. You want them about the size and thickness of the coin.
4. Drop into your pitcher and add in the mango.
5. Top with 3 cups of ice and then add with water.(the ice is important, it holds down the ginger and mango to help infuse the water)
6. Place in your fridge for 1-3 hours before serving.
7. When serving add a couple frozen mango chunks in a pretty glass for ice cubes.

Detox Lemon and Lime Water

Ingredients

- ✓ 1 lemon
- ✓ 3 lime
- ✓ Ice cubes
- ✓ Water

Directions

- ✓ Slice the lemon and lime, and add to a pitcher or jug. Top up with water, and pop in the fridge to cool down. Once it's cold, add ice and serve! Ah, the freshness!

Notes

- ✓ You can vary how much lemon and lime you add, some like more, some want less flavour

Dieter's Dream Water

For a richer approach to detoxifying, you cannot surpass the diverse qualities of this renowned recipe. While it relies on the industry standard of lemon and cucumber, this is clearly only just the start.
***Servings:* 1**

Ingredients
- ✓ Large pitcher of cold filtered water
- ✓ 1 lemon thinly sliced
- ✓ ½ cucumber thinly sliced
- ✓ Small bunch cilantro (stems cut off)
- ✓ Small bunch Italian parsley (stems cut off)
- ✓ Handful of frozen cranberries

Directions
1. Mix all ingredients together and refrigerate.
2. I make mine the night before so the flavour from the ingredients is stronger.
3. Continue to refill with water for throughout the day.

Ginger Orange Water

This is also an amazing metabolism booster. It is chock full of Vitamin C, which is an immunity booster. Ginger again is effective for soothing an upset tummy. This infused water aids your health and gives your weight loss a boost.

Ingredients
- ✓ ½ an orange
- ✓ 1 to 1.5 inch strip of ginger

Directions

- ✓ Add the peeled and sliced ginger in a jug. Add orange slices to this and squeeze a few of the orange slices. Top it with water and let it steep for up to an hour.

Lemon Berry Fat Flush Water

Lemon Berry Fat Flush is perfect for the summer to keep you hydrated and to flush out those bad toxins in your body. Drink up to 8-10 cups daily to help maintain a flat tummy.

Servings: 1

Ingredients

- ✓ 1/2 cup blueberries, fresh or frozen
- ✓ 1/2 cup raspberries, fresh or frozen
- ✓ 1 lemon, sliced
- ✓ 3 cups water, purified

Directions

- ✓ Add all ingredients to a large glass, cover with lid and allow to chill overnight in the refrigerator, drink throughout the day. Most importantly enjoy that fresh taste.

Lemon Berry Flush Fat Spa Water

If you want to implement a stricter regimen, then you should dabble with this lively lemon water detox.

Servings: 1

Ingredients

- ✓ 1/2 cup blueberries, fresh or frozen
- ✓ 1/2 cup raspberries, fresh or frozen

✓ 1 lemon, sliced

✓ 3 cups water, purified

Directions

✓ Add all ingredients to a large glass, cover with lid and allow to chill overnight in the refrigerator, drink throughout the day.

Lemon Blackberry Infused Water

Ingredients

✓ 1/4-1/2 lemon, washed and sliced (I really love lemon so I use 1/2)

✓ 5-6 blackberries, washed

Directions

✓ Combine lemon, blackberries and ice. Add 16 oz. water. Screw on the lid and give it a few good shakes. Refrigerate 4-24 hours. Muddle the berries with the back of a spoon or fork, enjoy!

Lemon Cucumber Refresher

Ingredients

✓ 1/2 lemon to 1 lemon , sliced very thinly

✓ 1/2 cucumber, sliced very thinly

✓ Ice, as required

✓ 2 liters water

Directions

✓ Add the lemon and cucumber to a jug, and top it with water and ice. Let it steep for a minimum of an hour. You can store it up to 24 hours.

Master Cleanse Detox Water

Ingredients & Directions:

This master cleanse detox water recipe is designed to flush every bad toxin out of your body. You will need about twelve ounces of filtered water, 2 tablespoons of lemon juice, 2 tablespoons of organic maple syrup, 1/10 of a teaspoon of cayenne pepper and a dash of sea salt. Just mix the ingredients together and drink. There are also optional ingredients like green tea and laxatives that you can add but the detox water in itself is great for ridding your body of free radicals and leaving you feeling and looking much healthier.

Orange-Kiwi Infused Water

Ingredients

- ✓ 2 cups of water or sparkling water
- ✓ 2 cups of ice
- ✓ 1 orange, sliced
- ✓ 2 kiwis, peeled and sliced

Directions

- ✓ Combine all in a large mason jar or jug and drink immediately or let sit in fridge for 1-4 hours to soak in additional flavor.

Peppermint Grapefruit Detox Water

A refreshing pitcher of water filled with fresh fruit that will help detoxify your body.
Servings: 1 | Prep: 5 m | Ready In: 5 m

Ingredients

- ✓ ½ gallon purified water
- ✓ ½ lemon, sliced
- ✓ ½ lime, sliced
- ✓ ½ grapefruit, sliced
- ✓ 1 cup cucumber, sliced
- ✓ 1 tsp ginger, sliced (add more if you like)
- ✓ A small handful of peppermint leaves

Directions

1. In a large picture add all of your ingredients and give it a mix. Add some ice cubes if you like. Place in the refrigerator for at least 2 hours before drinking. Discard the water after 24 hours if you don't drink it all.
2. Recipe slightly modified from Skinny Mommy

Nutrition Information

- • Serves: 8 cups
- • Serving size: 1 cup

Notes

- ✓ Please be sure not to drink it after 24 hours, as the fruit tend to get soggy, strong tasting from the citrus.
- ✓ Also, you can also add sliced oranges if you like.
- ✓ No calories in this drink! Drink as much as you like and enjoy!

Pineapple Jalepeno Lemon Infused Water

Ingredients

- ✓ 1/8 pineapple, cut into tidbits
- ✓ 1/4-1/2 lemon, washed and sliced (also great without it)
- ✓ Jalapeno, washed and cut into 4 thin slices, membranes and seeds removed (wear gloves when cutting)

Directions

1. Add pineapple to the jar and muddle, then add lemon, and jalapeno. Add ice and water, screw on the lid and give it a good shake. Enjoy immediately! You can also refill your jar a few times or dilute it with more water if it's too spicy to start.
2. And speaking of canning jars...click each pic for details!

Pineapple Sugarcane Spa Water

Ingredients & Directions

If you prefer a bit of a tropical taste in your detox water, this pineapple and sugarcane water is perfect. The pineapple helps to rid your body of free radicals and this recipe is so easy that you can make it in about five minutes. You need a couple of liters of purified water, 2 sticks of sugar cane and a few chunks of fresh pineapple. Note, fresh works much better than canned. Just mix all of the ingredients in a pitcher and add ice. Let it steep in the fridge for a couple of hours before drinking. The longer it sits, the better it tastes.

Pomegranate Tarragon Water

This slightly sweet and herbal detox water is an easy way to up your daily water intake. If you start with a whole pomegranate you'll have extra seeds to use for another batch!
Servings: 4-6 | **Prep:** 10 m | **Cook:** 30 m | **Ready In:** 40 m

Ingredients

- ✓ 1 pomegranate or ¼ cup pomegranate seeds
- ✓ ¼ cup fresh tarragon
- ✓ 1 quart water

Directions

1. If using a whole pomegranate there is a little trick to removing the seeds that will make the experience much more pleasant.

2. Roll the fruit on a cutting board with the back of your hand to loosen the seeds slightly.

3. Score the top with an x and tear the pomegranate open with your hands.

4. Submerge the pomegranate into a large bowl of water and push the edges down and away to loosen the fruit. Using a large wooden spoon, tap the skin with a wooden spoon to release the rest of the fruit. Remove any of the pith that floats to the top, and drain the water.

5. Measure out ¼ cup of the seeds and save the rest for another use.

6. Place the pomegranate seeds into a small bowl and use the back of a wooden spoon or muddler to lightly smash the seeds and release the juice. Alternatively, if you have a mortar and pestle you can use that to smash the seeds. Add the seeds and tarragon to a large pitcher and fill with the water. Let sit for at least 30 minutes or overnight before drinking.

Raspberry Orange Water

Ingredients
- ✓ 2 cups fresh raspberries
- ✓ 2 oranges
- ✓ 2 quarts water

Directions
1. Add raspberries to a jar or pitcher and break up gently with a wooden spoon.

2. Cut the oranges into wedges; squeeze juice into the jar and then toss the wedges in too.
3. Add water, cover, and chill until ready to serve.

Strawberry Kiwi Slimdown Water

Kiwi detox water belongs to a league of its own. This exotic fruit is blessed with tons of dietary fiber, which helps it remove extra sodium from the system. Girls who consume too much salt may discover a lot of assistance through these tropical treats.

Servings: 1 | Prep: 5 m | Cook Time: 15-20 m

Ingredients
✓ ½ gallon cold water
✓ 2 kiwis, sliced
✓ 6 strawberries, sliced

Directions
1. Serving size: ½ gallon
2. Mix all ingredients and keep chilled.
3. Allow the ingredients to chill in the refrigerator for 1-2 hours before serving. Discard after 24-48 hours or when fruit starts to taste bitter.
4. *The recipe is meant to be drank without eating the fruit itself.
5. Tip: You can get the daily recommended 8 glasses of water by drinking this entire recipe throughout the day!

Strawberry Mango Water–Skin

Servings: 4

Ingredients
- ✓ 1 cup of fresh, ripe mango - cubed
- ✓ 1/2 cup fresh strawberries - quartered
- ✓ 2 quarts of water
- ✓ Ice

Directions
1. Add mango cubes, strawberry quarters (about 6 strawberries) to a pitcher. Cover with water and let steep in the refrigerator for about 4 hours.
2. Serve over ice for a subtle fragrant fresh beverage!

Notes
- ✓ The fruit swells from the water. If serving more than 8 hours from the time you make it, I recommend replacing the fruit in the pitcher with fresh fruit for a more visual appealing presentation.

Strawberry Spa Water

This summertime drink feels so luxurious and refreshing, you'll think you're in your own home spa. It's perfect for brunches or baby showers, or just to get some extra antioxidants. Whip up a pitcher when strawberries go on sale!

Yields: *4-6 glasses*

Ingredients
- ✓ 1 lb strawberries, hulled and sliced
- ✓ 1 pitcher filtered water
- ✓ Ice

Directions
1. Add strawberries and water to pitcher. Cover and refrigerate for at least 6 hours or up to overnight.
2. Add ice just before serving. Enjoy!

Vegan Strawberry Lemonade

Strawberries, raspberries, and squeezed lemons infused overnight make the best vitamin water! Color hydrate your body!

Ingredients
- ✓ 4-5 sliced strawberries
- ✓ Handful ripe raspberries
- ✓ 2 sliced lemons

Directions
- ✓ Slice all ingredients as desired and place into your jar. Fill your glass with water, then place in the refrigerator overnight or until chilled. The longer that you let it sit, the more the colors will melt into the water, creating a pink lemonade! Enjoy in the sunshine!

Watermelon Detox Water

What better fruit to add to your water than watermelon? Not only does watermelon contain vitamins and minerals, it helps to flush out your system. Instead of eating it and making that juicy and sticky mess, just add a bit to your water to enjoy the full detoxing benefits.

Ingredients
- ✓ 2 cups Seedless Watermelon, cubed
- ✓ 4 cups Water

Directions
1. Place Watermelon in pitcher and cover with Water.
2. Let it sit a few hours in the refrigerator before drinking - so the water gets all the nice watermelon flavor.

Sparkling - Based Recipes
* * *

10-Minute Sparkling Watermelon Limeade

Easy and healthy, turn your favorite summer fruit into a refreshing drink in under 10 minute!
Servings: 4 | Total time: 15 m

Ingredients
- ✓ 4 cups/32 ounces cubed seedless watermelon
- ✓ Juice of 2-3 seeded limes (or lemons), preferably organic
- ✓ Liquid honey or agave syrup (according to your taste)
- ✓ Sparkling water

Directions
1. Blend the watermelon until smooth. Add the lime juice, honey or agave syrup and blend again.
2. Pour into a punch bowl and add sparkling water to taste, or until you get the desired consistency.
3. Pour into glasses over ice —you can strain the juice before serving, if you like, but I did not find it necessary. Keep cool in a sealed container and drink quickly.

Aperol Spritz

Servings: 1 | Total time: 10 mins

Ingredients
- ✓ Ice
- ✓ Orange slice
- ✓ 3 parts Prosecco

- ✓ 2 parts Aperol
- ✓ 1 part sparkling water

Directions

- ✓ Add ice and a slice of orange to a glass. Pour in the Prosecco, then the Aperol, and finally the sparkling water. This order prevents the Aperol from settling at the bottom.

Blood Orange Rosemary Sparkling Water

Servings: 4 | Total time: 15 mins

Ingredients

- ✓ 2 tablespoons honey
- ✓ 3 tablespoons water
- ✓ 4 small sprigs rosemary, divided
- ✓ 3 large blood oranges (enough for 1 cup juice)
- ✓ 750 mL sparkling water (we use the soda maker shown here)

Directions

1. Heat 2 tablespoons honey, 3 tablespoons water and 3 sprigs rosemary over low heat for about 1 minute until fully combined. Allow to cool on the stove, and then discard the rosemary.
2. Juice 3 blood oranges. In a pitcher, combine the honey mixture, orange juice, and sparkling water. Garnish with the remaining rosemary sprig and serve.

Cucumber Melon Sangria

Servings: 5 | Total time: 25 mins

Ingredients

- ✓ 1 (750 ml) bottle dry white wine
- ✓ 3/4 cup gin
- ✓ 2 tablespoons superfine sugar
- ✓ 1/2 honeydew melon, cubed
- ✓ 1/2 seedless cucumber, sliced
- ✓ 1/2 cup packed fresh mint leaves
- ✓ 1 cup sparkling water or club soda

Directions

1. Combine all ingredients except sparkling water in a large pitcher and still well. Refrigerate at least 3 hours (more if possible).
2. Just before serving, pour in sparkling water and gently stir to combine. Serve over ice.

DIY Sparkling Beverage

Servings: 6 | Total time: 15 mins

Ingredients

- ✓ 2-3 (32 ounce) bottles sparkling water (I use Apollinaris)
- ✓ 1 (32oz) bottle fruit juice (I used pineapple, though anything would work)

Directions

1. Partially fill some fancy glasses 2/3 full with sparkling water
2. Top with fruit juice
3. Garnish with lemon, lime or orange slices
4. Serve

Healthy Sparkling Fruit Water

It's been so hot here, and every day my kids and I are trying to come up with new ways to keep cool. I decided to freeze some pomegranate juice and blueberries and combine it in sparkling lime-flavored water to create this super refreshing and healthy Sparkling Fruit Water. It's so easy!
Servings: *4* | **Prep:** *10 mins*

Ingredients

- ✓ 1 (8-ounce) bottle pomegranate juice
- ✓ 5 cups lime-flavored sparkling water, divided
- ✓ 1/2 cup fresh blueberries
- ✓ 1 lime, thinly sliced

Directions

1. Pour pomegranate juice in ice cube trays. Pour 2 cups lime-flavored sparkling water in another ice cube tray. Add blueberries in the trays with sparkling water. Freeze at least 8 hours or overnight.
2. Pour remaining sparkling water in a pitcher. Remove ice cubes from trays and serve immediately.

Nutritional Information

- ✓ Calories77
- ✓ Fat0.2 g (0.4%)
- ✓ Saturated0 g (0.1%)
- ✓ Carbs14.3 g (4.8%)
- ✓ Fiber0.6 g (2.5%)
- ✓ Sugars11.1 g
- ✓ Protein1 g (2%)
- ✓ Sodium40.6 mg (1.7%)

Mojito

Servings: *2* | **Total time:** *5 mins*

Ingredients

- ✓ 40 ml White Rum
- ✓ 30 ml Fresh lime juice
- ✓ Slice lime
- ✓ 6 Sprigs of mint
- ✓ 2 teaspoon brown sugar
- ✓ Sparkling water
- ✓ Ice cubes

Directions

- ✓ Put the mint leaves on one hand and clap. This bruises the leaves and releases the aroma. Add brown sugar and four lime wedges into a highball glass and muddle. Fill a highball glass with crushed ice and add white rum. Top off with sparkling water and slice of lime. Garnish with slice of lemon and spring of mint.

Orange Creamsicle Sparkling Water

Servings: 4 | Total time: 10 mins

Ingredients

- ✓ ½tsp Vanilla
- ✓ 1tsp Orange Extract
- ✓ 1 slice of orange
- ✓ Sparkling Water

Directions

1. Fill a glass with ice.
2. Add vanilla and orange extract.
3. Add sparkling water and stir.
4. If desired, squeeze orange slice into water or use for a garnish.

Passionfruit Sparkling Mineral Water

Servings: 2 | Prep: 1 mins | Total time: 10 mins

Ingredients
- ✓ 2 passion fruit
- ✓ 2 glasses cold sparkling mineral water
- ✓ Sweetener of choice (optional)

Directions
- ✓ Cut open the passion fruit and add to glasses. Pour on the sparkling water and mix with the sweetener if you're having some.

Pineapple & Strawberry Sangria

Servings: 5 - 6 | Prep: 15 mins | Total time: 15 mins

Ingredients
- ✓ ½ pineapple cut into ½" to 1" pieces
- ✓ 1½ cup sliced strawberries
- ✓ juice from 1 lemon
- ✓ 1 cup grape juice
- ✓ 1 bottle sparkling water with no sugar
- ✓ ¼ cup agave (or adjust accordingly to suit your taste)
- ✓ 10-12 mint leaves (optional)
- ✓ ice cubes for serving
- ✓ 1 lemon sliced

Directions
1. In a medium bowl muddle pineapple pieces and then transfer into a pitcher.

2. Add grape juice, lemon juice, sliced strawberries and mint leaves. Give it a mix. Refrigerate the mixture till serving.
3. Before serving add chilled sparkling water, lemon slices and adjust sweetness if necessary. Serve with ice cubes to beat the heat!

Notes

✓ When you have optimally ripe fruits you will not need to add additional sweetener.

Pineapple Mint Infused Sparkling Lime Water

Total time: 15 mins

Ingredients

✓ 6 large chunks of fresh pineapple
✓ 1 can of DASANI® Sparkling Lime Water
✓ 1 sprig of mint

Directions

1. Place the chunks of pineapple into an 8-ounce glass.
2. Pour the DISANI® over the pineapple, then add the sprig of mint.
3. Allow the drink to sit for just a short while to let the flavor of the mint set in.

Raspberry Shrub

Serving: 1 | Total time: 10 mins

Ingredients

✓ 3 tablespoons Simple Syrup
✓ 2 tablespoons Raspberry Vinegar (Click for recipe)

- ✓ 1 tablespoon brandy (optional)
- ✓ Sparkling water or Prosecco
- ✓ Lemon slice
- ✓ Mint sprig

Directions

- ✓ Stir simple syrup, raspberry vinegar, and brandy (optional) in a 12-ounce glass. Fill glass halfway with ice. Fill glass with sparkling water or Prosecco. Garnish with a lemon slice and a mint sprig.

Sparkling Basil Lemonade

Ingredients

- ✓ 4 cups water
- ✓ 3 cups sugar
- ✓ 2 cups fresh basil leaves (about 1-1/2 ounces)
- ✓ 2 1 liter bottles club soda, chilled
- ✓ 2 cups lemon juice
- ✓ Ice cubes
- ✓ 1 fresh jalapeno chile pepper, sliced*
- ✓ Fresh basil leaves

Directions

1. For basil syrup, in a large saucepan combine water, sugar, and basil. Bring to boiling over medium-high heat. Reduce heat. Simmer, uncovered, for 20 minutes. Strain syrup and discard leaves. Cover and chill syrup for 2 to 24 hours.
2. For lemonade, in a very large punch bowl combine chilled syrup, club soda, and lemon juice. Serve over ice and garnish with jalapeno slices and fresh basil leaves.

Sparkling Berry Soda

*Servings: 12 | **Prep**: 5 mins | **Total time**: 5 mins*

Ingredients

- ✓ 2 cups frozen mixed berries
- ✓ 1 cup water
- ✓ 1/2 cup sugar
- ✓ Carbonated water, club soda, seltzer

Directions

1. Add all ingredients to the blender and blend on low-medium variable speed for 2-3 minutes.
2. Strain resulting mixture (berry simple syrup) through fine mesh sieve/strainer.
3. Add ice to glass with 1 ounce of berry simple syrup t and fill with carbonated water, club soda or seltzer.
4. Add additional berry simple syrup to taste.

Notes

- ✓ I like to use a frozen berry mix of blueberries, strawberries, raspberries and blackberries.

Sparkling Cherry Lemonade

*The easiest, budget-friendly lemonade that you can make in just 15 min.
No simple syrup needed!*
*Servings: 6 | **Prep**: 15 mins | **Total time**: 15 mins*

Ingredients

- ✓ 12 ounces cherries, pitted
- ✓ 3/4 cup freshly squeezed lemon juice
- ✓ 2/3 cup sugar
- ✓ 4 cups sparkling water

Directions

1. To make the cherry syrup, combine cherries, lemon juice and sugar in blender until smooth. Place in the refrigerator until chilled.
2. Serve over ice and sparkling water.

Sparkling Cherry Limeade Water

*Servings: 1 | **Prep**: 5 mins | **Total time**: 5 mins*

Ingredients

✓ 100% Cherry Juice*
✓ Fresh Limes
✓ Sparkling Key Lime Water
✓ Born Sweet® Zing™ Zero Calorie Stevia Sweetener

Directions

1. Fill up a glass 3/4ths the way full with pebble or crushed ice.
2. Pour the cherry juice to fill the glass 1/4th the way full. Fill up another 1/4th with freshly squeezed lime juice. (Equal parts cherry and lime juice)
3. Fill up the remainder of the glass with sparkling key lime water.
4. Add in 1-2 packets of Born Sweet® Zing™ Zero Calorie Stevia Sweetener. Garnish with a slice of lime if desired.
5. Enjoy immediately.

Notes

✓ Check the ingredients to ensure there is ONLY Cherry juice (no added filtered water or other juices) to get the strongest cherry flavor.

Sparkling Cherry Smoothie

Serving: 4 | Total Time: 10 mins

Ingredients

- ✓ 1/2 lb cherries (fresh, pitted, plus extra to decorate)
- ✓ 1/4 lb strawberies, hulled
- ✓ 1/8 lb blueberries
- ✓ 8 ice cubes
- ✓ 12/3 cups sparkling mineral water
- ✓ Mint sprigs (fresh, to serve, optional)

Directions

- ✓ Place cherries and the berries in a blender or food processor and process until smooth. Divide between four chilled glasses, add a couple of ice cubes to each glass and top up with sparkling mineral water. Decorate with mint sprigs and whole cherries, if desired.

Sparkling Citrus Coconut Water

A refreshing drink recipe made with citrus and sparkling coconut water
Servings: 4 | Prep: 5 mins | Total time: 5 mins

Ingredients

- ✓ 1 grapefruit
- ✓ 2 lemons
- ✓ 2 oranges
- ✓ 3 limes
- ✓ 1 liter naturally flavored pineapple coconut sparkling water

Directions

- ✓ Start by slicing all the citrus fruits. Squeeze some of the juice into a large pitcher and put in the slices. Pour in 1 liter of naturally flavored pineapple coconut sparkling water and stir. Pour into glasses filled with ice cubes and garnish with citrus slices.

Sparkling Grape Juice-Lemonade

Freeze grapes in clusters as purchased. This is not a girl's-only punch; it's a hit with men too.

Yield: *Makes 4 servings*

Ingredients

- ✓ 1 bunch seedless grapes (about 1/3 lb.)
- ✓ 1 (750-milliliter) bottle sparkling white grape juice, chilled
- ✓ 1/4 cup thawed frozen lemonade concentrate

Directions

1. Place grapes in a zip-top plastic freezer bag; seal bag. (Do not remove grapes from stems.) Freeze completely (about 4 hours).
2. Gently stir together grape juice and lemonade concentrate in a large pitcher. Add frozen grapes to pitcher. Serve immediately.

Note

- ✓ Grapes may be stored in freezer up to 1 week. For photography we doubled the recipe.

Sparkling Immunity Juice

This pleasantly fizzy drink may taste like a fruity cocktail, but it is

seriously good for you! Drink it to keep your immune system strong year round. And drink it because it tastes gosh darn delicious.
***Servings**: 2 | **Prep**: 10 mins | **Total time**: 10 mins*

Ingredients

- 2 cups freshly squeezed orange juice
- 1 inch knob ginger
- 1 inch knob turmeric
- 2 teaspoons honey, optional
- 1 cup sparkling water (more or less to taste)

Directions

1. Combine the orange juice, ginger, turmeric, and honey in a blender. Blend until smooth.
2. Strain the juice through a fine mesh sieve or piece of cheesecloth. Pour into glasses and top each glass with desired amount of sparkling water.

Sparkling Kiwi Lemonade Recipe

Yield: 6 servings

Ingredients

- ✓ 8 medium kiwifruit, peeled, divided
- ✓ 3/4 cup sugar
- ✓ 3/4 cup lemon juice
- ✓ 1 liter carbonated water, chilled

Directions

1. Slice two kiwi into small pieces. Place in ice cube trays and fill with water. Freeze.
2. Cut remaining kiwi into large pieces; place in a food processor. Cover and process until smooth. Strain; discard pulp. In a 2-qt. pitcher, stir sugar and lemon juice

until sugar is dissolved. Stir in kiwi puree. Refrigerate until chilled. Just before serving, stir in carbonated water. Serve over kiwi ice cubes.

Sparkling Mango Lemonade

Refreshing and delightful sparkling pulpy lemonade made with mangoes and agave.
***Servings**: 2 | **Prep**: 5 mins | **Total time**: 5 mins*

Ingredients

- ✓ 1 1/2 cup Frozen Mango Chunks (I like Wyman's, gotta support local business!)
- ✓ 1 1/2 cup Lemonade (I like Newman's Own)
- ✓ 1/2 cup Sparkling Water or Club Soda
- ✓ 2 teaspoons Agave Nectar

Directions

1. Add mango, lemonade, and agave to a blender and blend until liquid.
2. Add sparkling water or club soda and give it a light pulse.
3. Pour into sugar rimmed glasses and garnish with a lemon wedge.

Sparkling Mint Lemonade

The ultimate summer quencher, lemonade is refreshing as it is, but can be wonderfully lightened with sparkling water and fresh mint. The result is a nonalcoholic punch similar to a mojito.
***Servings**: 12 | **Total time**: 15 mins*

Ingredients

- ✓ 1 cup fresh mint leaves, plus more for garnish

- ✓ 8 fl. oz. simple syrup (see note above)
- ✓ 1 cup fresh lemon juice
- ✓ 6 cups cold water
- ✓ Ice, as needed
- ✓ 2 cups sparkling water
- ✓ Lemon wheels for garnish

Directions

- ✓ In a punch bowl, combine the mint leaves and simple syrup. Using a muddler or wooden spoon, gently muddle the mint leaves, being careful not to tear them. Stir in the lemon juice and cold water. Add ice and the sparkling water. Garnish with lemon wheels and mint leaves. Makes 12 drinks.

Notes

- ✓ To make simple syrup, in a measuring cup, stir together 1/4 cup superfine sugar in 1/4 cup hot water until dissolved. Let cool. This recipe makes 3 fl. oz. syrup and can be doubled or tripled as needed.

Sparkling Mint Melon Limeade

Servings: 4 | Prep: 10 mins | Total time: 10 mins

Ingredients

- ✓ 1/4 cup fresh squeezed lime juice
- ✓ 2 1/2 cups chopped or cubed honeydew melon
- ✓ 2 cups sparkling water or flavored sparking water (lime, lemon, ginger etc.)
- ✓ 2 mint leave sprigs
- ✓ Sliced lime for pitcher or garnishing
- ✓ 1/4 cup honey or maple syrup (agave works too)

✓ Stevia or xylitol if you want it sweeter without the added sugar

Directions

1. First make sure your fruit it cut. I would slice up one lime for garnishing and the other for juicing. Next, blend together your honey dew, water, and 2 -3 mint leaves. Save a few leaves for garnishing.
2. Pour water melon mix into a pitcher. Add your honey or sweetener, lime juice, and extra lime slices/mint leaves.
3. If you want more fizz, add in more sparkling water.
4. IF you want it sweeter, add in stevia or xylitol and adjust to your liking.

Notes

✓ Substitutes To make sweeter you can use a flavored sparkling water or even zevia (natural diet soda).
✓ Works well with cantaloupe melon too!

Sparkling Mint Peach Lemonade

*Servings: 3 | **Prep**: 3 hours | **Total time**: 3 hours*

Ingredients

✓ 32 ounces of water
✓ 2 packets of CRYSTAL LIGHT On the Go Lemonade flavor
✓ 2/3 cup peach nectar
✓ Handful of mint leaves
✓ Splash of sparkling water

Directions

1. In a large pitcher, fill with 32 ounces of cold water. Pour the lemonade packets in and stir to mix well. Add the peach nectar and stir to combine.

2. Using the end of a wooden spoon, muddle the mint leaves when added to the pitcher to release some of its minty flavor. You can remove the mint leaves after this or keep them in there for decoration.
3. Place pitcher in the refrigerator and chill for 2-3 hours, or until cold.
4. Pour into glasses and add a generous splash of sparkling water. Serve and enjoy!

Sparkling Mojito Water

*Servings: 4 | **Prep**: 5 mins | **Total time**: 10 mins*

Ingredients
- ✓ 6 TBS Fresh Lime Juice {about 2 limes}
- ✓ 4 TBS Stevia in the Raw {or other sweetener}
- ✓ 8 Mint Leaves
- ✓ 36 ounces Sparkling Water

Directions
1. Juice limes.
2. Muddle mint and lime juice. That means stick the mint in the lime juice and crush it around to release the oils.
3. Stir in sweetener.
4. Move to a larger container and add sparkling water.
5. Serve over ice and garnish with a lime wedge and sprig of mint.
6. Or just drink it all yourself. That's Ok, too.

Sparkling Peachy Punch

"This is a beautiful, tasty punch that is simple to make. Frozen peaches makes this punch stand out on the table. All liquid should be cold before

starting!"
*Servings: 24 | **Prep**: 10 m | **Ready In**: 10 m*

Ingredients

- ✓ 1 (64 fluid ounce) bottle chilled white cranberry-peach juice (such as Ocean Spray® White Cran-Peach)
- ✓ 1 liter chilled lemon-lime soda (such as Sprite®)
- ✓ 2 (11.5 ounce) cans peach juice, chilled, or to taste
- ✓ 2 (10 ounce) packages frozen peach slices
- ✓ 1 (12 ounce) package frozen raspberries (optional)

Directions

- ✓ Mix white cranberry juice, lemon-lime soda, and peach juice together in a punch bowl. Float as many peach slices and raspberries in the punch as desired. Place remaining fruit back in freezer and add as needed.

Cook's Note

- ✓ Start with one can peach juice and add the second to your taste of sweetness.

Nutritional Information

- ✓ Calories:86 kcal 4%
- ✓ Fat: 0 g < 1%
- ✓ Carbs: 21.1g 7%
- ✓ Protein: 0.4 g < 1%
- ✓ Cholesterol: 0 mg 0%
- ✓ Sodium: 10 mg < 1%

Sparkling Punch

"Sparkling apple cider, fresh orange juice, and lemonade concentrate blend into light and refreshing non-alcoholic punch in this easy recipe."
*Servings: 24 | **Prep**: 10 m | **Ready In**: 10 m*

Ingredients
- ✓ 2 lemons
- ✓ 3 large oranges
- ✓ 1 (6 ounce) can frozen lemonade concentrate
- ✓ 1 liter club soda
- ✓ 2 (750 milliliter) bottles sparkling apple cider
- ✓ 1 tablespoon white sugar
- ✓ 2 trays ice cubes

Directions
- ✓ Thinly slice the lemons and the oranges and place in a large punch bowl. Pour in the thawed lemonade. Gently stir in the club soda and the sparkling apple cider. Add sugar to taste. Add ice.

Nutritional Information
- ✓ Calories: 73 kcal 4%
- ✓ Fat: 0.1 g < 1%
- ✓ Carbs: 18.9g 6%
- ✓ Protein: 0.4 g < 1%
- ✓ Cholesterol: 0 mg 0%
- ✓ Sodium: 11 mg < 1%

Sparkling Raspberry Lemonade

Servings: 5 | Total time: 35 mins

Ingredients
- ✓ ½ cup water
- ✓ ½ cup granulated sugar
- ✓ 6 ounces fresh raspberries
- ✓ 1 cup freshly squeezed lemon juice (about 7 to 8 lemons)
- ✓ 3 ½ cups cold sparkling water

Directions

1. Start by making a simple syrup to sweeten the lemonade. In a small saucepan, add the ½ cup water and ½ cup granulated sugar. Heat over medium high, stirring occasionally, until the sugar has completely dissolved. Remove from the heat and set aside to cool slightly.

2. Add the raspberries to the bowl of a food processor. Process until smooth. Strain the raspberry puree through a fine mesh sieve to remove the seeds (using a wooden spoon to help push it through).

3. In a large pitcher or container, add the raspberry puree and lemon juice. Pour in the simple syrup (If you are not sure how sweet you want the lemonade, start with some of the syrup - you can always add more later. I used all of the syrup). Mix to combine. Right before serving, add in the sparking water and mix gently to combine (you can store the mixture in the refrigerator until you are ready to serve and then just add the sparkling water at the last minute).

Sparkling Rum Mojito

Servings: 4 | Total time: 10 mins

Ingredients

- ✓ 10 fresh mint leaves
- ✓ 1/2 lime, cut into 3-4 slices
- ✓ 2 tablespoons white sugar
- ✓ 1 1/2 cup ice cubes
- ✓ 1 1/2 fluid ounces rum
- ✓ 1/2 cup Vintage Sparkling Water

Directions

1. Place crushed mint leaves and squeeze the juice of one lime slice into glass, top with ice. Add other ingredients to a martini shaker with 1/2 cup of ice and shake to mix. Pour over ice, garnish with mint and enjoy!

2. *Check out the product locator page to find Vintage Sparkling Water in a store near you. A 12-pack of sparkling water typically retails $3.99.

Sparkling Smashed Raspberry Mint Lemonade

Servings: 6 | Total time: 10 mins

Ingredients

- ✓ 12 ounces fresh raspberries
- ✓ 1 cup raw honey
- ✓ ½ cup water
- ✓ 1 cup fresh lemon juice
- ✓ Ice
- ✓ 1 liter sparkling mineral water
- ✓ 6 fresh mint leaves, cut into fine ribbons, plus more for garnish
- ✓ Lemon slices, for garnish

Directions

1. Place raspberries in a bowl and smash with a whisk.

2. In a medium bowl, mix together honey, water and lemon juice. Add smashed raspberries and mint ribbons.

3. For each serving, place half a cup of raspberry honey lemon juice mixture in a glass. Fill glass with ice. Add sparkling mineral water to the brim. Stir and garnish with mint sprig and lemon slice.

Sparkling Strawberry Lemonade Refresher

Sugar free sparkling strawberry lemonade is the perfect mix of sweet and crisp with a hint of tartness that's perfect for warm sunny days.
Servings: *5 - 6* | **Total time**: *35 mins*

Ingredients

- ✓ 1½ cups ripes strawberries
- ✓ ½ cup erythritol (I used Swerve)
- ✓ 3 lemons
- ✓ 24 oz sparkling water (I used Perrier lemon)

Directions

1. In a medium bowl muddle pineapple pieces and then transfer into a pitcher.
2. Add grape juice, lemon juice, sliced strawberries and mint leaves. Give it a mix. Refrigerate the mixture till serving.
3. Before serving add chilled sparkling water, lemon slices and adjust sweetness if necessary. Serve with ice cubes to beat the heat!

Notes

- ✓ When you have optimally ripe fruits you will not need to add additional sweetener.

Sparkling Strawberry Lemonade

Wonderfully sweet, tangy, refreshing and bubbly. Plus, it's so easy and inexpensive to make right at home!

Ingredients

- ✓ Lemons - 6
- ✓ Sugar Syrup - 1+1/2 cup

- ✓ Strawberries - 1 cup hulled
- ✓ Sparkling water or club soda - 1 liter
- ✓ Ice cubes
- ✓ Lemon wedges for garnishing

Directions

1. Combine ¾ cup of sugar and ¾ cup of water in a pan and bring to a boil. Stir until sugar has dissolved and then let it cool down completely.
2. Microwave lemons for 15 seconds to release the juices. Cut the lemons in half and juice into a bowl. Remove any seeds. You will get about 1 cup of lemon juice.
3. Blend the strawberries with sugar syrup until smooth.
4. Pour lemon juice, strawberry puree, and sparkling water into a pitcher. Add ice cubes and chill until ready to drink.
5. Place more ice cubes in a glass and pour in chilled lemonade. Garnish with lemon wedges and Enjoy!

Sparkling Strawberry Peach Sangria

This fresh, fruity sangria will make any weekend a party! Perfectly fizzy and bubbly with plenty of juicy peaches and strawberries.
***Servings**: 8 | **Prep**: 10 mins | **Total time**: 10 mins*

Ingredients

SIMPLE SYRUP:

- ✓ 5 cups peeled and sliced fresh peaches, divided
- ✓ 5 cups halved fresh strawberries, divided
- ✓ 1/2 cup water
- ✓ 2/3 cup xylitol (or sugar)
- ✓ *SANGRIA*
- ✓ 1-1/2 cups white wine

✓ 1-1/2 cups sparkling water

Directions

1. Make the simple syrup: Place 4 cups peaches, 4 cups strawberries, water, and xylitol (or sugar) in a medium saucepan. Bring to a boil over medium-high heat, stirring occasionally until fruit is broken down and soft. Remove from heat and cool.

2. Press mixture, a little at a time through a mesh sieve, discarding solids (or saving for another use) Transfer remaining juice to a serving pitcher. Stir in wine, sparkling water, and remaining 1 cup peaches and 1 cup strawberries. Chill sangria in refrigerator until cold.

Notes

✓ If you wish to make this sangria completely fresh and no-cook, feel free to use freshly squeezed juice in the place of the simple syrup. (if you're looking for a great juicer, check out these awesome ones) Simply omit the simple syrup and use 2 cups of fresh juice instead.

Sparkling Strawberry Water

Servings: 2 | Prep: 1 m | Cook: 1 m | Ready In: 2 m

Ingredients

✓ 6 to 10 strawberries
✓ 2 glasses sparkling mineral water

Directions

1. Crush 1 or 2 strawberries per person and slice up the rest.

2. Mix with the water in a glass and hydrate

Sparkling Watermelon Cucumber Coolers

Serving: 4 | Total time: 35 mins

Ingredients
- ✓ 2 cups fresh watermelon juice
- ✓ 1 (12 ounce) can Vintage Sparkling Cucumber Melon Water
- ✓ 1 cup fresh watermelon chunks
- ✓ 6 cucumber slices

Directions
1. To make watermelon juice combine 4 cups of watermelon chunks in a blender and blend until smooth, pour through a mesh strainer. This should give you 2 cups of fresh watermelon juice.
2. To make the Sparkling Cucumber Melon Coolers divide the melon and cucumber among two glasses and fill with ice. Combine the juice and sparkling water in a small pitcher, stir to combine. Pour the Sparkling Cucumber Melon juice in the glasses.
3. Serve immediately.
4. To make larger servings just use 2 cups of watermelon juice for each can of Vintage Sparkling Cucumber Melon Water you use.

Sparkling Watermelon Lemonade

Servings: 8 | Total time: 15 mins

Ingredients
- ✓ 1 12 oz. can frozen lemonade concentrate
- ✓ 4 heaping cups cubed seedless watermelon

- ✓ 6 cups chilled lemon lime soda
- ✓ (If you prefer things a little less sweet, consider using sparkling water instead)
- ✓ Ice

Directions

- ✓ Blend watermelon in blender until smooth. Pour watermelon into a pitcher and add lemonade concentrate, stirring until combined. Slowly add the chilled soda and stir. Add ice and garnish with lemon slices (optional) and enjoy! Best if served immediately or store leftover sparkling watermelon lemonade covered in the refrigerator.

Sparkling Watermelon Limeade

Servings: 5 | Total time: 25 mins

Ingredients

- ✓ 1 cup water
- ✓ 1 cup sugar
- ✓ 1 cup ice
- ✓ 6 cups diced watermelon, pureed and strained {should yield 3 1/2 cups watermelon juice}
- ✓ 2/3 cup freshly squeezed lime juice
- ✓ 2 cups sparkling water {such as Perrier or S.Pellegrino}
- ✓ ice
- ✓ extra watermelon pieces or lime wedges for garnish, if desired

Directions

In a small saucepan, bring water and sugar to boil until sugar is dissolved. Remove from heat and stir in ice to cool quickly. Pour simple syrup into pitcher with watermelon juice, lime juice and sparkling water. Stir and serve over ice with watermelon and lime wedges.

Recipe note

✓ Depending on how sweet your watermelon is, you may need to add more or less simple syrup as required.

Sparkling Watermelon Mocktail

Servings: 1 | Total time: 10 mins

Ingredients

✓ 1/2 cup watermelon cubes
✓ 8 ounces lemon/lime or plain seltzer or sparkling water
✓ 1/4 packet sugar free lemonade mix (preferably sweetened with stevia)

Directions

1. Muddle watermelon in a glass.
2. Add seltzer and lemonade mix.
3. Stir gently- the powdered mixure will fizz in the seltzer at first.
4. optional: add a shot of vodka, rum or other favorite alcohol
5. Thread extra watermelon cubes onto a straw for garnish if desired.

Notes

✓ If you prefer a less sweet beverage, simply add 1-2 teaspoons of lemon juice instead of the powdered lemonade mix.

Nutritional Information

✓ 24 calories
✓ 1g fat
✓ 1g sat fat

- ✓ 1mg sodium
- ✓ 5.8g carbohydrate
- ✓ 3g fiber
- ✓ 5g sugar
- ✓ 5g protein

Sparkling Watermelon Sangria

*Servings: 4 to 6 | **Total time**: 30 mins*

Ingredients

- ✓ 4 cups watermelon, cubed and cold
- ✓ 3/4 cups dry white port, such as Churchill's
- ✓ 1 lime, sliced thin
- ✓ 750ml bottle Moscato, chilled*
- ✓ 3 cups lime seltzer water, chilled

Directions

1. In a pitcher place 3 cups of the watermelon cubes (saving some for garnish) and white port. Be sure these are cold as they can become mushy when room temp. (You can even freeze them for 30 minutes first.)
2. Add 8 to 10 slices of lime.
3. Add the Moscato and seltzer water. Stir with wooden spoon to mix.
4. Pour into ice-filled glasses and top each glass with a couple pieces of watermelon and a lime slice.
5. Wine recommendation: I like 7 Daughters Moscato because it's delicious and not too sweet, and it's under $15/bottle.

Nutritional Information

- ✓ Calories: 77
- ✓ Fat: 0.2 g (0.4%)

- ✓ Saturated: 0 g (0.1%)
- ✓ Carbs: 14.3 g (4.8%)
- ✓ Fiber: 0.6 g (2.5%)
- ✓ Sugars: 11.1 g
- ✓ Protein: 1 g (2%)
- ✓ Sodium: 40.6 mg (1.7%)

Sparkling Watermelon Sippers

Total time: 15 mins

Ingredients
- ✓ 1/2 cup white grape juice (I used Welch's)
- ✓ 2 cups watermelon
- ✓ 1 cup sparkling water

Directions
- ✓ Combine watermelon and grape juice in a blender, and blend until smooth. Â In a glass, pour watermelon juice till the glass is half full. Â Top off the glass with sparkling water.

Sparkling Watermelon Slushie

What's better than a slushie? A SPARKLING Watermelon Slushie that won't mess up your clean eating lifestyle because it's simply perfect.
Yields: 2

Ingredients
- ✓ 2 cups frozen seedless watermelon chunks
- ✓ About ½ can of berry-flavored sparkling water like La Croix or Canada Dry
- ✓ Juice of one lime (or lemon juice if you're in a pinch)

Directions
1. If the watermelon has been in the freezer for more than 2 hours, allow to thaw a bit at room temperature (just to soften for the blender, not thaw completely)
2. Add watermelon, lime juice and sparkling water (a little at a time) to the blender and mix well.

Stone Fruit and Ricotta Picnic Plate

Servings: 9 | **Prep**: 10 mins | **Total time**: 10 mins

Ingredients
Stone Fruit and Ricotta Crisps
- ✓ 2 pounds of assorted stone fruit (white nectarines, apricots, pluots, yellow plums, etc.)
- ✓ 15-ounces whole milk ricotta cheese
- ✓ 1 cup raw unsalted walnuts
- ✓ ¼ cup fresh mint leaves
- ✓ 34 Degrees Whole Grain Crisps

Additional Picnic Supplies

✓ Knives and spoons

✓ Sparkling water with mint and lemon

✓ Castelvetrano olives

✓ Additional cheeses, meats, etc.

Directions

1. Juice limes.
2. Prepare a picnic board with ripe stone fruits, ricotta cheese, walnuts, mint, and crisps.
3. Create a simple pairing by topping a whole grain crisp with a dollop of ricotta, a slice of fruit, a piece of walnut and a mint leaf.

Strawberry Hibiscus Sparkling Water

This is my new favorite flavored water recipe! This strawberry hibiscus sparkling water is so refreshing and perfect for summer.

***Servings**: 8 | **Prep**: 5 mins | **Total time**: 2 h 5 mins*

Ingredients

✓ 1 cup fresh strawberries

✓ 2 tablespoon dried hibiscus flowers

✓ 2 16.9 oz bottles sparkling water

Directions

1. Slice strawberries and place in a pitcher.
2. Add dried hibiscus flowers.
3. Pour one bottle of sparkling water over the strawberries and hibiscus flowers. Refrigerate for a couple hours.
4. Pour second bottle of sparkling water into pitcher right before serving.
5. Enjoy!

Strawberry Lemon Sparkling Water

Strawberry Lemon Sparkling Water is an easy sparkling water recipe that will keep your body hydrated and your tastes buds happy!
***Servings**: 1 | **Prep**: 5 mins | **Total time**: 5 mins*

Ingredients
- ✓ 1 liter plain sparkling water
- ✓ 6-8 strawberries, sliced
- ✓ 1-2 drops therapeutic grade lemon essential oil (I use Young Living) or 3-4 fresh lemon slices

Directions
- ✓ Add strawberries, lemon oil or slices to sparkling water. Gently move the bottle in a circular motion. Let chill in refrigerator at least 2 hours. Serve with ice if desired.

Strawberry Mojito Sparkling Water

A light and refreshing summer drink, this strawberry mojito mocktail is made with lime sparkling water and fresh herbs and berries.
***Servings**: 1 | **Prep**: 5 mins | **Total time**: 5 mins*

Ingredients
- ✓ 1 can Lime Vintage Sparkling Water
- ✓ 5 Strawberries, sliced
- ✓ 4-5 Mint leaves
- ✓ 2 Lime slices
- ✓ Ice

Directions
1. Put 4 sliced strawberries and mint leaves in a glass and crush them until the fruit is broken up and the leaves are bruised.

2. Add ice to glass.
3. Pour lime Vintage sparkling water over ice.
4. Add lime slices and the last of the strawberry slices to the drink.
5. Garnish with fresh mint and a strawberry.

Strawberry Orange Spritzer

Servings: 4 | Total time: 15 mins

Ingredients
- ✓ 8 oz. sparkling mineral water
- ✓ 2 tsp Terre Exotique Orange Water
- ✓ drizzle of honey of sprinkle or Nektar Naturals honey crystals (to taste)
- ✓ strawberries
- ✓ mint leaves (for garnish)

Directions
1. Mix together mineral water, orange water and honey until dissolved.
2. Add sliced strawberries and mint leaves.
3. Garnish glass with a strawberry!

Tito's All-Time Favorite

Servings: 4 | Total time: 5 mins

Ingredients
- ✓ 1 1/2 oz Tito's Handmade Vodka
- ✓ 4 oz sparkling mineral water
- ✓ Slice of orange
- ✓ Slice of lime

Directions

- ✓ Combine Tito's Handmade Vodka and mineral water into cocktail glass with ice. Stir and garnish.

Tom Collins

*Servings: 4 | **Prep**: 1 mins | **Total time**: 5 mins*

Ingredients

- ✓ 45 ml Gin
- ✓ 15 ml Simple syrup
- ✓ 30 ml Fresh lemon juice
- ✓ 60 ml Sparkling water
- ✓ Orange slice and cherry

Directions

- ✓ Fill a cocktail shaker with ice. Add gin, fresh lemon juice and simple syrup. Shake and strain into a highball glass with ice cubes. Top off with sparkling water and add slice of orange. Garnish with slice of orange and cherry.

Triple Berry Sparkling Natural Fizzy Water

*Yield: 3 - 4 cups of fizzy water | **Prep Time**: 10 mins*
Total Time: 15 mins

Ingredients

- ✓ 1 cup blueberries
- ✓ 1 cup raspberries
- ✓ 1 cup strawberries
- ✓ 2 cups Perrier Sparkling Water
- ✓ *Optional*
- ✓ honey to sweeten

✓ strainer

Directions

✓ Blend blueberries, raspberries and strawberries with 1 cup Perrier Sparkling Water in a blender.

✓ Pour in the pitcher and add another 1 cup Perrier Sparkling Water.

Optional

✓ You can sweeten the fizzy water with honey and also if you don't like fruits in the water use strainer to separate the fruits from the water.

Tropical Sparkling Water

Servings: 8 | Prep: 10 mins | Total time: 10 mins

Ingredients

✓ 8 - 12 oz. cans Dasani Sparkling Tropical Pineapple

✓ assorted fruit (I used grapes, pineapple, and kiwi!)

✓ 1 lemon, optional

Directions

1. Fill 8 highball glasses half-full with ice.
2. Place about ⅓ c. cut-up assorted fruit into the glass.
3. Spritz with a touch of fresh lemon juice.
4. Fill glass with Dasani Sparkling Tropical Pineapple.

Ultimate Sparkling Fruit Punch

Servings: 7 | Total time: 15 mins

Ingredients

✓ 1 lb fresh strawberries, stems removed and halved

✓ ¼ cup fresh blueberries (44 g)

- ✓ ½ cup fresh black grapes (90 g)
- ✓ ½ cup freshly squeezed lemon juice (do not use that pre-made stuff at the store!)
- ✓ 4-6 tablespoons pure maple syrup (I only used 4 tablespoons but feel free to adjust, I found this to be just enough sweetness to cut the bitter and not be too sweet)
- ✓ 4 cups sparkling water, chilled

Note:

- ✓ It is important your sparkling water is chilled for several hours or overnight because if you add it room temperature and then chill the drink afterwards, the carbonation will fizz out by the time you serve it. To save time, you can have all your fruit ready the day before and then just add everything a few minutes before serving to your blender when it's all nice and cold.

Directions

1. Before starting, make sure your sparkling water has chilled for a long time in the fridge (see above note).
2. Wash all your fruit and chop the strawberries and remove stems. Add them along with all the remaining ingredients to a blender and blend until completely smooth. Taste and add any more sweetener if desired. I find this was plenty sweet with 4 heaping tablespoons, but if you are serving it at a party, you may add a little more.
3. Lastly, drain the punch through a fine mesh strainer to catch any skins left behind from the grapes. See above photo in post. It does catch a lot. Pour in a pitcher and over ice if desired and serve. I garnished my glasses with extra fruit.

Two: Detox Juice

***

Lemonade Recipes

* * *

Amy's Cucumber Lemonade

"Refreshing summer sipping drink. I had this drink at a local restaurant and liked it so much I had to re-invent it in my own kitchen. Serve over ice."

Servings: 6 | Prep: 5 m | Ready In: 5 m

Ingredients

- ✓ 1 (6 ounce) can frozen lemonade concentrate
- ✓ 4 (6 ounce) cans water
- ✓ 1 cucumber, peeled and sliced

Directions

- ✓ Place lemonade concentrate into a jug with a lid and stir in 3 lemonade cans of water. Pour 1 more can of water into a blender, add cucumber, and puree. Pour cucumber mixture into lemonade and shake to thoroughly mix.

Nutritional Information

- ✓ Calories:70 kcal 4%
- ✓ Fat: 0.1 g < 1%
- ✓ Carbs: 18g 6%
- ✓ Protein: 0.3 g < 1%
- ✓ Cholesterol: 0 mg 0%
- ✓ Sodium: 6 mg < 1%

Basil Lemonade

"I tweaked this recipe it to make a refreshing drink. I love basil and this

recipe has a wonderful basil-infused flavor. Delicious on a warm day or with grilled chicken. Serve over ice and garnish with fresh basil and lemon slices."

*Servings: 12 | **Prep**: 15 m | **Ready In**: 8 h 10 m*

Ingredients

- ✓ 12 cups cold water
- ✓ 1 (12 ounce) can frozen lemonade concentrate, thawed
- ✓ 1/3 cup white sugar
- ✓ 1/4 cup fresh lime juice
- ✓ 1/2 cup firmly packed torn basil leaves

Directions

- ✓ Stir water, lemonade, sugar, and lime juice together in a pitcher. Add 1/2 cup basil leaves, stir to combine, cover the pitcher, and refrigerate until flavors combine, 8 hours to overnight. Remove basil leaves and discard.

Cook's Note

- ✓ Add or subtract the preferred amount of lemonade concentrate for stronger or weaker lemonade flavor. Substitute bottled lime juice for fresh lime juice.

Nutritional Information

- ✓ Calories:89 kcal 4%
- ✓ Fat: 0.1 g < 1%
- ✓ Carbs: 23.2g 7%
- ✓ Protein: 0.2 g < 1%
- ✓ Cholesterol: 0 mg 0%
- ✓ Sodium: 9 mg < 1%

Best Strawberry Lemonade Ever

"Strawberry lemonade is a very refreshing drink and this is my version of the best one ever! So refreshing on a hot summer day! Serve chilled."

Servings: 6 | Prep: 15 m | Cook: 5 m | Ready In: 35 m

Ingredients

- ✓ 12 fresh strawberries, hulled and quartered
- ✓ 1/4 cup white sugar
- ✓ 7 cups water, divided
- ✓ 3/4 cup white sugar
- ✓ 1 cup lemon juice
- ✓ 2 cups ice cubes

Directions

1. Mix strawberries and 1/4 cup sugar together in a bowl; set aside for juices to release from strawberries, 5 to 10 minutes.

2. Bring 1 cup water to a boil in a small saucepan; add 3/4 cup sugar. Cook and stir sugar mixture until sugar is dissolved, about 5 minutes. Remove saucepan from heat and cool simple syrup to room temperature.

3. Stir simple syrup, 6 cups water, lemon juice, and ice together in a pitcher. Add sweetened strawberries and stir.

Cook's Note

- ✓ I always mix the ice and simple syrup together first and give it a good stir so that the syrup is nice and cold before I add the remaining ingredients.
- ✓ Remove seeds from lemon juice, but leave pulp.

Nutritional Information

- ✓ Calories:151 kcal 8%
- ✓ Fat: 0.1 g < 1%
- ✓ Carbs: 39.6g 13%
- ✓ Protein: 0.4 g < 1%
- ✓ Cholesterol: 0 mg 0%
- ✓ Sodium: 11 mg < 1%

Bethy's Cucumber Basil Lemonade

"I make this refreshing lemonade all summer long. It goes great at any picnic!" **Servings**: 8 | **Prep**: 15 m | **Cook**: 5 m | **Ready In**: 2 h 15 m

Ingredients

- ✓ 8 cups cold water, divided
- ✓ 1 cup white sugar
- ✓ 1 1/2 cups lemon juice
- ✓ 1/2 cucumber, thinly sliced
- ✓ 10 fresh basil leaves, torn

Directions

1. Combine 1 cup water and sugar together in a small saucepan; bring to a boil. Cook and stir until sugar is dissolved, about 5 minutes. Remove saucepan from heat and cool syrup to room temperature.
2. Stir syrup, remaining water, lemon juice, cucumber, and basil together in a pitcher; chill in the refrigerator for at least 2 hours.

Nutritional Information

- ✓ Calories:110 kcal 6%
- ✓ Fat: 0 g < 1%
- ✓ Carbs: 29.4g 9%
- ✓ Protein: 0.3 g < 1%
- ✓ Cholesterol: 0 mg 0%
- ✓ Sodium: 8 mg < 1%

Chia Fresca

"This is a refreshing drink much like lemonade."
Servings: 12 | **Prep**: 5 m | **Ready In**: 15 m

Ingredients

- ✓ 1 1/2 cups water
- ✓ 3 tablespoons lemon juice
- ✓ 2 1/2 teaspoons white sugar
- ✓ 1 teaspoon chia seeds

Directions

- ✓ Stir water, lemon juice, and sugar together in a glass until sugar is completely dissolved; add chia seeds. Let stand until a gel forms around the chia seeds, about 10 minutes; stir.

Nutritional Information

- ✓ Calories:64 kcal 3%
- ✓ Fat: 0.8 g 1%
- ✓ Carbs: 15.4g 5%
- ✓ Protein: 0.6 g 1%
- ✓ Cholesterol: 0 mg 0%
- ✓ Sodium: 12 mg < 1%

Citrus Lemonade

"So simple, so refreshing. What more do you need?"
Servings: 12 | **Prep**: 20 m | **Ready In**: 20 m

Ingredients

- ✓ 1 cup white sugar, or to taste
- ✓ 4 lemons, juiced
- ✓ 4 limes, juiced
- ✓ 4 oranges, juiced
- ✓ 3 quarts cold water
- ✓ 1 lime, sliced into rounds (optional)
- ✓ 12 cups ice cubes

Directions

✓ Pour the sugar, lemon juice, lime juice, and orange juice into a gallon-sized container; stir until the sugar has dissolved. Serve over ice with a slice of lime if desired.

Nutritional Information

✓ Calories:107 kcal 5%

✓ Fat: 0.2 g < 1%

✓ Carbs: 30.2g 10%

✓ Protein: 1.2 g 2%

✓ Cholesterol: 0 mg 0%

✓ Sodium: 16 mg < 1%

Easy Brazilian Lemonade

"This drink is SOO good!"
*Servings: 3 | **Prep**: 10 m | **Ready In**: 10 m*

Ingredients

✓ 2 limes

✓ 3 cups water

✓ 1/2 cup white sugar

✓ 3 tablespoons sweetened condensed milk

✓ 1 cup ice cubes

Directions

1. Wash limes thoroughly. Cut ends off and discard, then slice into about 8 pieces.

2. Place limes, water, sugar, and sweetened condensed milk in a blender. Pulse 5 times. Strain mixture through a sieve into a large pitcher. Serve over ice.

Nutritional Information

✓ Calories:203 kcal 10%

✓ Fat: 1.7 g 3%

- ✓ Carbs: 48.3g 16%
- ✓ Protein: 1.8 g 4%
- ✓ Cholesterol: 6 mg 2%
- ✓ Sodium: 34 mg 1%

Easy Lemonade

"You can use a combination of lemon and lime, or lemon and orange, or lemon, lime AND orange! 3/4 cup is about 3 large lemons, but measure it because you don't want it too tart!"

*Servings: 8 | **Prep**: 10 m | **Cook**: 5 m | **Ready In**: 15 m*

Ingredients

- ✓ 3/4 cup fresh lemon juice
- ✓ 2 quarts water
- ✓ 1/2 cup white sugar

Directions

- ✓ In a large pan, combine water and sugar. Heat until the sugar just melts. Remove from heat and pour in lemon juice. Mix well and chill in refrigerator before serving. Garnish with lemon, lime or orange slices.

Nutritional Information

- ✓ Calories:54 kcal 3%
- ✓ Fat: 0 g 0%
- ✓ Carbs: 14.5g 5%
- ✓ Protein: 0.1 g < 1%
- ✓ Cholesterol: 0 mg 0%
- ✓ Sodium: 7 mg < 1%

Fresh Lemonade

"A summer classic, this lemonade is easy and refreshing too!"

*Servings: 6 | **Prep**: 10 m | **Ready In**: 10 m*

Ingredients

- ✓ 10 lemons
- ✓ 3 cups water
- ✓ 2 cups white sugar
- ✓ 4 cups crushed ice

Directions

- ✓ Cut 1/2 of one lemon into thin slices and set aside. Juice remaining 9 1/2 lemons and pour into a glass pitcher or punch bowl. Stir in the water and sugar until dissolved. Pour in the crushed ice and float the lemon slices on top.

Nutritional Information

- ✓ Calories:294 kcal 15%
- ✓ Fat: 0.5 g < 1%
- ✓ Carbs: 85.9g 28%
- ✓ Protein: 2.2 g 4%
- ✓ Cholesterol: 0 mg 0%
- ✓ Sodium: 8 mg < 1%

Fresh Squeezed Lemonade with Truvia® Natural Sweetener

"Naturally refreshing! The tart bite of fresh squeezed lemons is balanced with the sweetness of Truvia® natural sweetener to quench your summertime thirst. This beverage has only 5 calories per serving."*
Serving: 2

Ingredients

- ✓ 1 3/4 cups chilled water
- ✓ 4 tablespoons fresh squeezed lemon juice (see note)
- ✓ 1 tablespoon Truvia® natural sweetener spoonable, plus

✓ 1/2 teaspoon Truvia® natural sweetener spoonable**

Directions

1. Combine ingredients and stir to dissolve.
2. Garnish rim of glass with fresh lemon slices or a strawberry, if desired. Serve over ice.

Gingerade

"Ginger ale and lemonade punch is an easy drink to make an is great at any party! You can use a cake pan to make an ice sculpture for your drink. When the water freezes, put the cake pan in a bowl of hot water for a few seconds, then put the ice in the punch bowl."

*Servings: 6 | **Prep**: 10 m | **Ready In**: 10 m*

Ingredients

✓ 2 (12 fluid ounce) cans or bottles ginger ale
✓ 1 cup granulated sugar
✓ 1 1/2 cups prepared lemonade
✓ 2 cups ice

Directions

✓ In a large punch bowl, combine the ginger ale, sugar, lemonade and ice. Stir to blend well and serve

Nutritional Information

✓ Calories: 195 kcal 10%
✓ Fat: 0 g < 1%
✓ Carbs: 49.8g 16%
✓ Cholesterol: 0 mg 0%
✓ Sodium: 19 mg < 1%

Jess' Party Punch

"Delicious but very dangerous cocktail for a group."

Servings: 8 | Prep: 5 m | Ready In: 5 m

Ingredients

- ✓ 1 (12 fluid ounce) can frozen pink lemonade concentrate, thawed
- ✓ 9 fluid ounces vodka
- ✓ 3 fluid ounces lemon-flavored rum (such as Bacardi Limon®)
- ✓ 1/2 lime, juiced
- ✓ 1 packet sugar substitute (such as Truvia®)
- ✓ 5 (12 fluid ounce) cans beer
- ✓ 32 ice cubes, or as desired

Directions

- ✓ Mix pink lemonade concentrate, vodka, rum, lime juice, and sugar substitute together in a pitcher. Add beer slowly; stir gently. Serve over ice.

Cook's Notes

- ✓ I prefer to use Budweiser(R) or Bud Light(R).
- ✓ Serve with caution, very delicious but very potent!

Nutritional Information

- ✓ Calories:292 kcal 15%
- ✓ Fat: 0.1 g < 1%
- ✓ Carbs: 34g 11%
- ✓ Protein: 1.2 g 2%
- ✓ Cholesterol: 0 mg 0%
- ✓ Sodium: 14 mg < 1%

Lavender Lemonade

"Enjoy this refreshing and soothing drink any time of the year."
Servings: 8 | Prep: 10 m | Cook: 5 m | Ready In: 30 m

Ingredients

- ✓ 2 cups boiling water
- ✓ 1 cup lavender flowers
- ✓ 2 cups cold water
- ✓ 1 cup lemon juice
- ✓ 1 cup sugar

Directions

- ✓ Place the lavender in a pitcher; pour the boiling water over the lavender; cover with plastic wrap and allow to steep 10 minutes; strain and discard the lavender from the water and return the water to the pitcher. Add the cold water, lemon juice, and sugar to the pitcher and stir until the sugar dissolves. Refrigerate until serving.

Nutritional Information

- ✓ Calories: 108 kcal 5%
- ✓ Fat: 0.1 g < 1%
- ✓ Carbs: 28.4g 9%
- ✓ Protein: 0.4 g < 1%
- ✓ Cholesterol: 0 mg 0%
- ✓ Sodium: 5 mg < 1%

Lemonade Plus

"This uses lemonade concentrate plus real fruit - lemons, limes, oranges, and grapefruit. It is soooo good."
***Servings**: 15 | **Prep**: 15 m | **Ready In**: 15 m*

Ingredients

- ✓ 2 (12 fluid ounce) cans frozen lemonade concentrate
- ✓ 1 lemon, sliced
- ✓ 1 lime, sliced
- ✓ 1 grapefruit, sliced

✓ 1 orange, sliced

Directions

✓ Into a gallon pitcher, empty both cans of lemonade concentrate. Place the sliced lemon, lime, grapefruit and orange in the pitcher. Stir in water until pitcher is full. Chill in refrigerator.

Nutritional Information

✓ Calories: 122 kcal 6%

✓ Fat: 0.2 g < 1%

✓ Carbs: 32g 10%

✓ Protein: 0.5 g 1%

✓ Cholesterol: 0 mg 0%

✓ Sodium: 3 mg < 1%

Malian Ginger Juice

"A popular and refreshing drink from West Africa. If it's too spicy, dilute with water. All ingredients can be adjusted to taste. This drink is great for cutting the heaviness of fried foods. Enjoy!"
Servings: 16 | **Prep**: 15 m | **Ready In**: 15 m

Ingredients

✓ 1/3 pound fresh unpeeled ginger root, cut into 1/2-inch chunks

✓ 1 1/2 cups water, or as needed to cover

✓ 4 large lemons, juiced

✓ 1 cup white sugar

✓ 7 cups water, or as needed

✓ 16 leaves fresh mint, crushed

Directions

1. Place ginger into a blender, cover with 1 1/2 cup water, and blend until ginger is thick and pasty. Strain and

squeeze juice from ginger pulp into a 2-quart pitcher, squeezing ginger mixture as dry as possible.

2. Stir lemon juice and sugar into ginger juice until sugar has dissolved. Pour 7 cups water into mixture, stir to combine, and serve garnished with crushed mint leaves.

Nutritional Information

- ✓ Calories:59 kcal 3%
- ✓ Fat: 0.1 g < 1%
- ✓ Carbs: 15.2g 5%
- ✓ Protein: 0.2 g < 1%
- ✓ Cholesterol: 0 mg 0%
- ✓ Sodium: 5 mg < 1%

Mason Jar Lemonade

"For those of us who want lemonade but want to make one serving of it. The perfect summer lemonade, still has the twang of lemon but lightly sweetened."

Servings: *1 |* ***Prep:*** *10 m |* ***Ready In:*** *10 m*

Ingredients

- ✓ 1 small lemon
- ✓ 1 1 quart mason jar
- ✓ 14 ounces cold water, divided, or to taste
- ✓ 1 1/2 tablespoons white sugar
- ✓ 5 ice cubes, or as needed

Directions

1. Roll lemon on a flat surface, cut in half, and squeeze juice and pulp into mason jar. Pour 12 ounces water into the jar.

2. Stir sugar and remaining 2 tablespoons water together in a small saucepan over medium heat until sugar dissolves. Pour sugar mixture and ice into mason jar and stir.

Cook's Notes

✓ Organic lemons are smaller in size than regular lemons you see in the store, so be careful as the ratio might be off. You may need to adjust the sugar amount to your personal preference.

Nutritional Information

✓ Calories:90 kcal 4%

✓ Fat: 0.3 g < 1%

✓ Carbs: 27.8g 9%

✓ Protein: 1 g 2%

✓ Cholesterol: 0 mg 0%

✓ Sodium: 18 mg < 1%

Meyer Lemonade with Mint

"Great for warm summer days."
*Servings: 6 | **Prep:** 15 m | **Ready In:** 2 h 15 m*

Ingredients

- 7 Meyer lemons, juiced
- 3 cups water
- 1/2 cup confectioners' sugar
- 1/4 cup chopped fresh mint

Directions

✓ Strain the lemon juice into a pitcher, and add the water, powdered sugar, and mint. Stir until the sugar has dissolved. Refrigerate at least 2 hours before serving.

Nutritional Information

✓ Calories: 67 kcal 3%

- ✓ Fat: 0.4 g < 1%
- ✓ Carbs: 24.4g 8%
- ✓ Protein: 1.6 g 3%
- ✓ Cholesterol: 0 mg 0%
- ✓ Sodium: 8 mg < 1%

Orangeade

"A refreshing change from lemonade. If you don't care for pulp in your drink, feel free to strain the juice before you add it to the water."
***Servings**: 8 | **Prep**: 5 m | **Cook**: 5 m | **Ready In**: 10 m*

Ingredients

- ✓ 2 cups water
- ✓ 1 1/2 cups white sugar
- ✓ 6 cups water
- ✓ 1 1/2 cups freshly squeezed orange juice
- ✓ 1/3 cup freshly squeezed lemon juice

Directions

1. Bring 2 cups water and sugar to a boil in a small saucepan; cook at a boil for 3 minutes, stirring to dissolve sugar, and creating a simple syrup.
2. Combine simple syrup, 6 cups water, orange juice, and lemon juice in a large pitcher; refrigerate until cold.

Nutritional Information

- ✓ Calories:169 kcal 8%
- ✓ Fat: 0.1 g < 1%
- ✓ Carbs: 43.2g 14%
- ✓ Protein: 0.4 g < 1%
- ✓ Cholesterol: 0 mg 0%
- ✓ Sodium: 8 mg < 1%

Peppermint Lemonade

"Cool, tingly, and oh so refreshing!"
***Servings**: 16 | **Prep**: 15 m | **Ready In**: 3 h 15 m*

Ingredients

- ✓ 1 (12 ounce) can frozen lemonade concentrate, thawed
- ✓ 1 fresh lemon
- ✓ 1 1/4 cups white sugar
- ✓ 1/2 cup fresh mint leaves

Directions

- ✓ Pour the lemonade concentrate into a large pitcher or cooler with a spout. Stir in enough water to make 1 gallon. Grate the zest from the lemon and add to the pitcher, then squeeze the lemon juice from the lemon into the pitcher. In a small bowl, crush the mint leaves into the sugar using a muddler or a wooden spoon. Stir into the lemonade. Cover and chill for several hours, then strain to remove the leaves and zest before serving. Serve over ice and garnish with a sprig of mint.

Nutritional Information

- ✓ Calories: 112 kcal 6%
- ✓ Fat: 0.1 g < 1%
- ✓ Carbs: 29.3g 9%
- ✓ Protein: 0.2 g < 1%
- ✓ Cholesterol: 0 mg 0%

Pineapple Lemonade Spritzers

"An alternative to lemonade, this summer cooler brings the flavor of the Mediterranean to you lips. Fresh mint leaves may be added for a twist."
***Servings**: 6 | **Prep**: 5 m | **Cook**: 5 m | **Ready In**: 1 d 10 m*

Ingredients

SYRUP:

- ✓ 3 cups pineapple juice
- ✓ 3 lemons, juiced
- ✓ 1 cup white sugar
- ✓ 1/2 cup honey
- ✓ 6 slices lemon
- ✓ 1 (2 liter) bottle carbonated water

Directions

1. To make the pineapple lemon syrup: In a large saucepan over medium heat, combine pineapple juice, lemon juice, sugar and honey. Bring to a boil, and cook for 1 minute. Allow to cool, then refrigerate overnight.
2. Fill 6 glasses with ice. Place a slice of lemon in each glass. Pour in 2 fluid ounces pineapple lemon syrup. Fill glasses to the top with carbonated water; stir.

Note

- ✓ The syrup can be stored in the refrigerator for up to 2 weeks.

Nutritional Information

- ✓ Calories: 295 kcal 15%
- ✓ Fat: 0.4 g < 1%
- ✓ Carbs: 79.9g 26%
- ✓ Protein: 1.3 g 3%
- ✓ Cholesterol: 0 mg 0%
- ✓ Sodium: 16 mg < 1%

Plantation-Style Vanilla Lemonade

"This lemon yellow lemonade is what I remember lemonade should taste like. Never watered down with a real lemon kick! Serve over ice or frozen

lemonade cubes."
*Servings: 6 | **Prep**: 10 m | **Ready In**: 10 m*

Ingredients
- ✓ 4 lemons
- ✓ 3/4 cup white sugar
- ✓ 1/4 teaspoon vanilla extract
- ✓ 6 cups cold water

Directions
- ✓ Cut the lemons in half and scoop the pulp into a blender. Add half of the rinds along with the sugar, vanilla extract, and 2 cups of the water. Blend until smooth, then strain into a serving pitcher and stir in the remaining water.

Nutritional Information
- ✓ Calories: 112 kcal 6%
- ✓ Fat: 0.2 g < 1%
- ✓ Carbs: 32.7g 11%
- ✓ Protein: 0.9 g 2%
- ✓ Cholesterol: 0 mg 0%
- ✓ Sodium: 9 mg < 1%

Quick Brazilian Lemonade

"Tasty lemonade with a creamy twist. I love this summertime treat, it hits the spot on hot days. Typically this drink is made with sweetened condensed milk, but using cream of coconut instead not only gives it more tropical flavor, but also makes it a dairy-free treat. Limes, not lemons you wonder? That is simply how Brazilian 'lemonade' is made."
*Servings: 6 | **Prep**: 10 m | **Ready In**: 10 m*

Ingredients
- ✓ 6 cups cold water

- ✓ 1 cup white sugar
- ✓ 4 limes
- ✓ 6 tablespoons cream of coconut

Directions

1. Stir water and sugar together in a bowl until sugar dissolves; chill in refrigerator.
2. Cut ends off of each lime and cut each lime into 8 segments.
3. Working in batches, pulse sugar-water and lime wedges together in a blender several times. Pour mixture through a strainer into a pitcher.
4. Stir cream of coconut into lime mixture.

Cook's Note

- ✓ Since this doesn't sit well, if you don't plan to serve this right away you can get the rest ready and refrigerate it until you are ready to mix in the cream of coconut and serve.
- ✓ Not familiar with cream of coconut? Look for it to be sold in cans around the mixed drink section since it is often used for pina coladas. Don't confuse with coconut cream; cream of coconut is much sweeter.

Nutritional Information

- ✓ Calories: 214 kcal 11%
- ✓ Fat: 3.4 g 5%
- ✓ Carbs: 49.1g 16%
- ✓ Protein: 0.3 g < 1%
- ✓ Cholesterol: 0 mg 0%
- ✓ Sodium: 18 mg < 1%

Radler

"Radler means 'cyclist' in German, and this refreshing drink was invented

*in Germany in the late 19th or early 20th century as a way to refresh
bicyclists worn out by the summer heat. It is a 50/50 or 60/40 mixture of
beer and lemonade and is a delicious addition to the menu of your
summer barbeque or party."*
Servings: 6 | **Prep**: 5 m | **Ready In**: 5 m

Ingredients
- ✓ 6 (12 ounce) cans pilsner-style beer, or to taste
- ✓ 2 quarts prepared lemonade, or to taste

Directions
- ✓ Combine beer and lemonade in a gallon-sized pitcher.

Cook's Notes
- ✓ Pilsner or lager work best for this drink, but feel free to experiment with your favorite. You'll need 1 to 2 six packs, depending on your taste.
- ✓ I prefer homemade lemonade, or Simply Lemonade(R) for a store-bought brand. You'll need one or two 1.75 liter bottles, depending on your taste.

Nutritional Information
- ✓ Calories: 285 kcal 14%
- ✓ Fat: 0.1 g < 1%
- ✓ Carbs: 47.1g 15%
- ✓ Protein: 1.9 g 4%
- ✓ Cholesterol: 0 mg 0%
- ✓ Sodium: 27 mg 1%

Refreshing Summer Cucumber Lemonade

*"This is the most refreshing summer beverage you've ever tasted. It's
unique in the way it infuses the flavors of fresh garden cucumbers, the
tangy brightness of fresh lemons, and the lightness of an effervescent
lemon-lime soda to create a delicious thirst quenching southern summer
ade. Perfect when relaxing on your front porch swing on a warm summer*

night."
*Servings: 6 | **Prep**: 15 m | **Ready In**: 45 m*

Ingredients

- ✓ 2 cups hot water
- ✓ 1/2 cup white sugar
- ✓ 1/2 cup lemon juice from concentrate
- ✓ 1 lemon, juiced
- ✓ 1/2 large cucumber, sliced
- ✓ 3 (12 fluid ounce) cans or bottles lemon-lime flavored soda
- ✓ 2 cups ice cubes, or as needed
- ✓ 1 lemon, thinly sliced
- ✓ 1/2 large cucumber, sliced and then halved

Directions

1. Stir hot water and sugar together in a large pitcher until sugar is dissolved. Stir in lemon juice concentrate, lemon juice, and sliced cucumbers. Refrigerate for 30 minutes or until ready to serve.
2. Pour lemon-lime soda into pitcher. Serve lemonade over ice and garnished with lemon slices and halved cucumber slices.

Nutritional Information

- ✓ Calories: 151 kcal 8%
- ✓ Fat: 0.1 g < 1%
- ✓ Carbs: 39.5g 13%
- ✓ Protein: 0.4 g < 1%
- ✓ Cholesterol: 0 mg 0%
- ✓ Sodium: 30 mg 1%

Rhubarb Lemonade

"A delicious pink rhubarb-flavored lemonade! To serve, mix 1 cup of rhubarb syrup with 3 cups of water and pour over ice."
Servings: 4 | **Prep**: 15 m | **Cook**: 10 m | **Ready In**: 25 m

Ingredients

- ✓ 8 cups chopped rhubarb
- ✓ 3 cups white sugar
- ✓ 3 tablespoons grated lemon peel
- ✓ 1 1/2 cups lemon juice

Directions

1. Combine the rhubarb, sugar, and grated lemon peel into a large saucepan and bring to a boil. Reduce heat to medium-low and simmer until the sugar has dissolved and the rhubarb releases its juice and starts to break up, about 10 minutes. Remove from heat and stir in the lemon juice.

2. Pour the rhubarb mixture through a fine sieve, pressing out as much liquid as possible.

Nutritional Information

- ✓ Calories: 657 kcal 33%
- ✓ Fat: 0.5 g < 1%
- ✓ Carbs: 169.7g 55%
- ✓ Protein: 2.6 g 5%
- ✓ Cholesterol: 0 mg 0%
- ✓ Sodium: 11 mg < 1%

Rosemary-Infused Watermelon Lemonade

"This is a recipe I created in an effort to duplicate my favorite lemonade from a cafe in downtown L.A. called, well, 'Lemonade'. I don't like it too sweet, so if you want to add more sugar, cool. But I think that this recipe is perfect. It also makes a great martini served in a sugar-rimmed glass

with a garnish of watermelon wedge and a twist of lemon! Simply fabulous!"

Servings: 8 | **Prep**: 15 m | **Cook**: 1 m | **Ready In**: 1 h 15 m

Ingredients

- ✓ 2 cups water
- ✓ 3/4 cup white sugar
- ✓ 1 sprig rosemary, leaves stripped and chopped
- ✓ 2 cups lemon juice
- ✓ 12 cups cubed seeded watermelon
- ✓ 8 cups ice cubes

Directions

1. Bring the water and sugar to a boil in a small saucepan over high heat. Stir in the rosemary, and set aside to steep for 1 hour.
2. Place half of the lemon juice, and half of the watermelon into a blender. Strain the rosemary syrup through a mesh strainer into the blender. Cover, and puree until smooth. Strain into a pitcher, then puree the remaining lemon juice and watermelon. Stir the lemonade before serving over ice.

Nutritional Information

- ✓ Calories: 156 kcal 8%
- ✓ Fat: 0.3 g < 1%
- ✓ Carbs: 41.2g 13%
- ✓ Protein: 1.6 g 3%
- ✓ Cholesterol: 0 mg 0%
- ✓ Sodium: 12 mg < 1%

Scorpion Lemonade

"Similar to the Master Cleanse Lemonade. Wonderful as part of a juice

cleanse. Caution: super spicy."
Servings: *1* | **Prep**: *5 m* | **Ready In**: *35 m*

Ingredients

- ✓ 14 fluid ounces water
- ✓ 3 fluid ounces lemon juice
- ✓ 1 tablespoon agave nectar
- ✓ 1/4 teaspoon cayenne pepper

Directions

- ✓ Combine water, lemon juice, agave nectar, and cayenne pepper in a bottle or jar with a lid; cover and shake well. Refrigerate until chilled.

Nutritional Information

- ✓ Calories: 84 kcal 4%
- ✓ Fat: 0.1 g < 1%
- ✓ Carbs: 24.2 g 8%
- ✓ Protein: 0.4 g < 1%
- ✓ Cholesterol: 0 mg 0%
- ✓ Sodium: 13 mg < 1%

Signature Sweet'N Low® Pink Lemonade

"Strawberries give this summer favorite a natural blush."
Servings: *1* | **Prep**: *10 m* | **Ready In**: *8 h 10 m*

Ingredients

- ✓ 1/4 cup fresh lemon juice
- ✓ 1/4 cup cold water
- ✓ 2 packets Sweet'N Low granulated sugar substitute
- ✓ 1 cup frozen strawberries, defrosted
- ✓ 1 lemon slice, for garnish (optional)
- ✓ 1 mint sprig, for garnish (optional)

Directions

1. In a large measuring cup, combine the lemon juice and water. Add the Sweet'N Low, stirring until it dissolves.
2. Spoon 1 tablespoon of liquid from the defrosted strawberries into a tall glass. Fill the glass with ice. Pour in the lemon juice mixture. If desired, garnish with the lemon slice and mint sprig. Enjoy the strawberries or save them for another use.

Cook's Note

✓ Defrosting frozen strawberries in the refrigerator takes 8 hours. Or defrost them at room temperature, about 1 hour. Defrosted berries keep in the refrigerator for 2 days.

Nutritional Information

✓ Calories:71 kcal 4%
✓ Fat: 0.2 g < 1%
✓ Carbs: 22.5g 7%
✓ Protein: 1.1 g 2%
✓ Cholesterol: 0 mg 0%
✓ Sodium: 6 mg < 1%

Spiced Lemonade Concentrate

"This old recipe for spiced lemonade is really delicious and refreshing. The spices really punch up the flavor and take it to the next level. To serve, pour 1 to 2 tablespoons of the concentrate into the bottom of a cup, add crushed ice, and mix with water, club soda, or ginger ale."
Servings: *8* | **Prep:** *10 m* | **Cook:** *20 m* | **Ready In:** *45 m*

Ingredients

✓ 1 cup water
✓ 1 cup white sugar

- ✓ 1 cinnamon stick
- ✓ 1/2 teaspoon whole cloves
- ✓ 1 lemon, juiced and zested
- ✓ 3 lemon, juiced

Directions

1. Combine water, sugar, cinnamon stick, cloves, and lemon zest in a saucepan; cook and stir over medium heat until just boiling, about 5 minutes.
2. Reduce heat to medium-low and continue to cook until reduced to a thick syrup, 10 to 15 minutes.
3. Stir lemon juice into the syrup; bring to a boil and cook 1 to 2 minutes more; strain into a bowl and refrigerate until chilled.

Nutritional Information

- ✓ Calories: 107 kcal 5%
- ✓ Fat: 0.1 g < 1%
- ✓ Carbs: 29.9g 10%
- ✓ Protein: 0.5 g 1%
- ✓ Cholesterol: 0 mg 0%
- ✓ Sodium: 3 mg < 1%

Tasty Lemonade

"This lemonade is good on hot days, and very successful at lemonade stands."

Servings: *4* | **Prep:** *15 m* | **Ready In:** *15 m*

Ingredients

- ✓ 6 lemons, juiced
- ✓ 1 1/2 cups water
- ✓ 1/2 cup brown sugar
- ✓ 1/2 cup ice cubes

Directions

- ✓ In a large pitcher, combine fresh lemon juice and water. Stir in brown sugar until it dissolves. Stir in ice cubes.

Nutritional Information

- ✓ Calories: 137 kcal 7%
- ✓ Fat: 0.5 g < 1%
- ✓ Carbs: 44.3g 14%
- ✓ Protein: 2 g 4%
- ✓ Cholesterol: 0 mg 0%
- ✓ Sodium: 13 mg < 1%

Thirst Quenching Lemonade

"Named after the golfer, it is said to be his favorite beverage.""This is a fantastic recipe which will quench your thirst. Once you try it, you will agree that this lemonade is better than lemonade you drink in a restaurant."

***Servings:** 2 | **Prep:** 5 m | **Ready In:** 5 m*

Ingredients

- ✓ 3/4 cup water
- ✓ 2/3 cup white sugar
- ✓ 4 fluid ounces lemon juice
- ✓ 1 1/4 cups ice water

Directions

1. In a saucepan, combine 3/4 cup water and 2/3 cup sugar. Bring to a boil and stir until sugar is dissolved. Set aside to cool. This step can be made in advance and stored in the refrigerator.
2. In a pitcher, combine syrup, lemon juice and ice water; stir. Adjust to taste. Pour into a tall glass with ice.

Nutritional Information

- ✓ Calories: 273 kcal 14%
- ✓ Fat: 0 g 0%
- ✓ Carbs: 71.9g 23%
- ✓ Protein: 0.2 g < 1%
- ✓ Cholesterol: 0 mg 0%
- ✓ Sodium: < 1 mg < 1%

More Detox Juice

*** *** ***

Agua Fresca de Pepino (Cucumber Limeade)

"This is another common agua fresca from Mexico. Refreshing, healthy, and delicious! Serve over ice."

Servings: 6 | **Prep**: 5 m | **Ready In**: 5 m

Ingredients

- ✓ 5 cups water, or to taste
- ✓ 3 cucumbers, peeled and chopped
- ✓ 1/2 cup freshly squeezed lime juice
- ✓ 1/4 cup granular sucralose sweetener (such as Splenda®), or to taste

Directions

- ✓ Blend 2 cups water, cucumbers, lime juice, and 2 tablespoons sweetener together in a blender until smooth. Pour into pitcher; add remaining water. Stir in additional sweetener to taste.

Nutritional Information

- ✓ Calories: 10 kcal < 1%
- ✓ Fat: 0 g < 1%
- ✓ Carbs: 4.4g 1%
- ✓ Protein: 0.1 g < 1%
- ✓ Cholesterol: 0 mg 0%
- ✓ Sodium: 6 mg < 1%

Apple Beet Juice

Yield: Makes 1

Ingredients

- ✓ 1 medium beet, chopped
- ✓ 1/2 lemon, chopped
- ✓ 3 stalks celery, chopped
- ✓ 2 sweet apples, chopped

Directions

- ✓ Press all ingredients through a juice extractor. Stir and serve immediately.

Apple Beetroot Carrot (ABC) Juice

Ingredients

- ✓ Carrot 1 medium
- ✓ Beetroot 1 medium peeled
- ✓ Apple 1 medium cored
- ✓ Orange 1 medium
- ✓ Celery stick 1 medium
- ✓ To serve
- ✓ Pink salt 1 tsp
- ✓ Lime juice 1 tsp
- ✓ Ice cubes a few (optional)

Directions

1. Juicer method:
2. If you have a juicer, then simply push all the veggies and fruits through the feeder and wait for the juicer to completely extract juice from the mixture.
3. Once done, add pink salt and 1 tsp of lime juice.
4. Mix well.
5. Drink the juice without straining.
6. Blender method:

7. You have to chop the apple, beet and carrot into cubes sized pieces before you place them in the blender.
8. Place the orange, beet, carrot, celery and apple in the blender along with the pink salt and lime juice. Add ½ c of water..
9. Blend to a smooth puree.
10. Strain and drink the juice immediately.

Banana Juice

"My husband taught me this recipe. It's yummy. Add a scoop of vanilla ice cream if you like (not to the blender, just on top)."
***Servings**: 2 | **Prep**: 10 m | **Ready In**: 10 m*

Ingredients
- ✓ 2 cups milk
- ✓ 2 large ripe bananas
- ✓ 2 tablespoons slivered shelled pistachios
- ✓ 1 tablespoon honey

Directions
- ✓ Blend milk, bananas, pistachios, and honey in a blender until smooth and frothy, about 2 minutes.

Cook's Notes
- ✓ Chill the bananas in the fridge beforehand for a colder drink.

Nutritional Information
- ✓ Calories: 320
- ✓ Calories:320 kcal
- ✓ Fat: 8.9 g
- ✓ Carbs: 53.3g
- ✓ Protein: 11.3 g
- ✓ Cholesterol: 20 mg

✓ Sodium: 136 mg

Beet, Apple, and Mint Juice

This healthy, invigorating juice will kickstart your morning.
Servings: 1

Ingredients
- ✓ 1 small beet, chopped
- ✓ 5 carrots, chopped
- ✓ 1 apple, cored and chopped
- ✓ 1/4 cup fresh mint sprigs

Directions
- ✓ Press beet, carrots, apple, and mint sprigs through a juice extractor. Stir and serve immediately.

Best Watermelon Slushie

"This is a healthy, delicious, refreshing treat for a hot day. Replace the honey with blue agave sweetener if you wish. Enjoy!"
Servings: 4 | Prep: 10 m | Ready In: 10 m

Ingredients
- ✓ 3 cups ice
- ✓ 2 cups watermelon chunks
- ✓ 1/2 cup cantaloupe chunks
- ✓ 1/4 cup orange juice
- ✓ 1 tablespoon honey
- ✓ 4 sprigs mint, for garnish (optional)

Directions
- ✓ Blend the ice, watermelon, cantaloupe, orange juice, and honey together in a blender until no chunks remain and

the mixture is a thick slush. Garnish with the mint if desired.

Nutritional Information

- ✓ Calories: 53 kcal 3%
- ✓ Fat: 0.2 g < 1%
- ✓ Carbs: 13.4g 4%
- ✓ Protein: 0.8 g 2%
- ✓ Cholesterol: 0 mg 0%
- ✓ Sodium: 10 mg < 1%

Black Grape-Purple Carrot Juice

Servings: 1 | Prep: 5 m | Ready In: 5 m

Ingredients

- ✓ 2 cups black or Concord grapes (12 ounces)
- ✓ 2 cups chopped purple carrots (10 ounces)

Directions

- ✓ Pass grapes and carrots through a juicer. Stir to combine; serve.

Blueberry Limeade

"Refreshing blueberry limeade is prepared with fresh blueberries, lime juice, and sugar. Serve cold over ice. Stir well before serving."

Servings: 8 | Prep: 5 m | Ready In: 5 m

Ingredients

- ✓ 2 cups fresh blueberries
- ✓ 1/2 cup white sugar, or to taste
- ✓ 1/3 cup freshly squeezed lime juice
- ✓ 6 cups water, or more as needed

Directions

- ✓ Blend blueberries, sugar, lime juice, and 1 cup water together in a blender; pour into a pitcher. Add remaining water and stir.

Nutritional Information

- ✓ Calories: 72 kcal 4%
- ✓ Fat: 0.1 g < 1%
- ✓ Carbs: 18.6g 6%
- ✓ Protein: 0.3 g < 1%
- ✓ Cholesterol: 0 mg 0%
- ✓ Sodium: 6 mg < 1%

Carrot and Apple Juice

"This is an extremely healthy drink I have almost every morning and great on detoxes as you get all your needed nutrients. You just have to play around to find the perfect drink. I find if you add beetroot, it makes it a fantastic color and gives extra flavor. To get the full benefit of the flavor, swish the juice around in your mouth; this is where lots of nutrients are digested. Enjoy!"

*Servings: 1 | **Prep**: 10 m | **Ready In**: 10 m*

Ingredients

- ✓ 4 carrots, trimmed
- ✓ 2 apples, quartered
- ✓ 2 stalks celery
- ✓ 1 (1/2 inch) piece fresh ginger

Directions

- ✓ Run carrots, apples, and celery through a juicer (alternating carrot, apple, and celery) according to manufacturer's instructions. Add ginger to juicer and process.

Nutritional Information
- ✓ Calories: 277 kcal 14%
- ✓ Fat: 1.3 g 2%
- ✓ Carbs: 68.6g 22%
- ✓ Protein: 4 g 8%
- ✓ Cholesterol: 0 mg 0%
- ✓ Sodium: 266 mg 11%

Carrot-Apple Juice

Carrot juice is surprisingly sweet, and goes well with the tartness of the apples. When buying Granny Smiths, choose firm ones; they will produce a clearer juice.

Servings: 1 | **Yield**: *Makes 10 Ounces*

Ingredients
- ✓ 3 or 4 medium carrots
- ✓ 1 medium Granny Smith apple
- ✓ Juicer

Directions
- ✓ Cut large produce into chunks, and remove big seeds or pits. Don't worry about those in fruits like apples and pears -- the juicer will filter them out. To combine several fruits and vegetables, alternate between soft pieces and hard ones. Finish with the latter to push through anything that's stuck.

Chai Limeade

"Get ready to spice up your summer with this extraordinary flavor combination even your kids will love. Sweet, tart, spicy, exotic and so easy to make. Great for brunches, pool-side, or sitting reading a book. Healthy

and flavorful. Serve over ice in coffee mugs for a feel of exotica!"
***Servings**: 2 | **Prep**: 10 m | **Ready In**: 15 m*

Ingredients

- ✓ 1 1/2 cups boiling water
- ✓ 3 chai tea bags, or more to taste
- ✓ 10 limes, juiced
- ✓ 1 lime, zested
- ✓ 4 cups ice, or as desired
- ✓ water, or as needed
- ✓ 1/4 cup white sugar, or to taste

Directions

1. Pour boiling water into a mug and add chai tea bags. Allow tea to steep for at least 5 minutes. Remove tea bags.
2. Combine lime juice and lime zest in a pitcher; add enough ice to fill pitcher halfway. Slowly pour chai tea over ice; stir. Add enough water to fill pitcher; stir in sugar.

Nutritional Information

- ✓ Calories: 50 kcal 3%
- ✓ Fat: 0 g < 1%
- ✓ Carbs: 14.1g 5%
- ✓ Protein: 0.3 g < 1%
- ✓ Cholesterol: 0 mg 0%
- ✓ Sodium: 13 mg < 1%

Cherry Sport Drink

"This drink is to be used in place of store-bought sport drinks filled with unrecognizable ingredients. Regular cherry juice can be used in place of tart cherry juice if desired. Coconut water can also be added."
***Servings**: 6 | **Prep**: 15 m | **Cook**: 5 m | **Ready In**: 4 h 15 m*

Ingredients

- ✓ 32 fluid ounces water
- ✓ 1 teaspoon sea salt
- ✓ 3 cups tart cherry juice (such as Knudsen®)
- ✓ 1/4 cup lemon juice

Directions

- ✓ Bring water and salt to a boil in a pot until salt is dissolved, 3 to 4 minutes. Stir cherry juice and lemon juice into salted water. Remove pot from heat and chill in refrigerator, about 4 hours.

Nutritional Information

- ✓ Calories: 73 kcal 4%
- ✓ Fat: 0.5 g < 1%
- ✓ Carbs: 17.4g 6%
- ✓ Protein: 0.5 g 1%
- ✓ Cholesterol: 0 mg 0%
- ✓ Sodium: 313 mg 13%

Citrus Blueberry Slush

"This recipe is super easy to make. Frozen orange juice and fresh blueberries are blended with ice to create a refreshing slush."
Servings: 4 | **Prep**: 5 m | **Ready In**: 5 m

Ingredients

- ✓ 1 (6 ounce) can frozen orange juice concentrate
- ✓ 6 fluid ounces water
- ✓ 1 cup fresh blueberries
- ✓ 4 cubes ice

Directions

- ✓ In a blender, combine orange juice concentrate, water, blueberries and ice cubes. Blend until slushy. Pour into glasses and serve.

Nutritional Information

- ✓ Calories: 105 kcal 5%
- ✓ Fat: 0.2 g < 1%
- ✓ Carbs: 25.6g 8%
- ✓ Protein: 1.5 g 3%
- ✓ Cholesterol: 0 mg 0%
- ✓ Sodium: 4 mg < 1%

Coconut Lemonade

Treat yourself to some coconut lemonade and allow yourself to be whisked away! Tropical umbrellas not included.

Ingredients

- ✓ 3 cups water
- ✓ 2/3 cup lemon juice
- ✓ 1/2 cup sugar
- ✓ 2 tablespoons coconut beverage flavoring syrup, such as Monin or Torani, or cream of coconut
- ✓ 1/2 cup frozen unsweetened blueberries
- ✓ 1/2 cup frozen red raspberries
- ✓ 1 small fresh carambola (star fruit), thinly sliced crosswise
- ✓ Ice cubes (optional)

Directions

1. In a large bowl combine water, lemon juice, sugar, and coconut syrup. Stir until sugar is well dissolved. Cover and chill for 4 to 24 hours.

2. To serve, transfer lemon mixture to a serving bowl or pitcher. Add blueberries, raspberries, and carambola. If desired, serve over ice cubes. Makes 4 (8-ounce) servings.

Colonial Holiday Cup

"Traditional hot, spiced beverage great for holiday gatherings or anytime when it's cold outside. You will find it superior to the powdered mixes. Continue to simmer and the spices will fill your home with a delightful aroma while keeping the beverage warm for continued enjoyment. "
Servings: 16 | Prep: 10 m | Cook: 1 h | Ready In: 1 h 10 m

Ingredients
- ✓ 1 gallon apple juice
- ✓ 1 cup orange juice
- ✓ 2 tablespoons lemon juice
- ✓ 6 cinnamon sticks
- ✓ 3/4 cup brown sugar
- ✓ 4 teaspoons whole cloves
- ✓ 2 teaspoons whole allspice
- ✓ 1 orange, sliced

Directions
- ✓ Pour apple juice, orange juice, and lemon juice into a large pot. Place the cinnamon sticks, brown sugar, cloves, and allspice onto the center of a 8 inch square piece of cheesecloth. Gather together the edges of the cheesecloth, and tie with kitchen twine to secure then add to the juice mixture. Float orange slices on top of the juices. Simmer over medium heat for 1 hour.

Nutritional Information
- ✓ Calories: 154 kcal 8%

- ✓ Fat: 0.4 g < 1%
- ✓ Carbs: 38.7g 12%
- ✓ Protein: 0.4 g < 1%
- ✓ Cholesterol: 0 mg 0%
- ✓ Sodium: 11 mg < 1%

Copycat V8® Juice

"Full of tomatoes, celery, onion, pepper, beet, carrot, and garlic, this vegetable juice cocktail tastes even better than the store-bought version!"
Servings: 4 | **Prep**: 20 m | **Cook**: 55 m | **Ready In**: 1 h 15 m

Ingredients

- ✓ 1 1/2 pounds tomatoes, chopped
- ✓ 1/3 large onion, chopped
- ✓ 3 tablespoons chopped celery
- ✓ 1/2 teaspoon chopped celery
- ✓ 3/8 carrot, chopped
- ✓ 1/4 beet
- ✓ 1/8 green bell pepper, seeded and chopped
- ✓ 1/3 clove garlic
- ✓ 2 1/3 cups water, or as needed
- ✓ 1 1/4 teaspoons white sugar
- ✓ 1 1/2 teaspoons lemon juice
- ✓ 1/4 teaspoon horseradish
- ✓ 1/4 teaspoon Worcestershire sauce, or to taste
- ✓ 1/8 teaspoon ground black pepper
- ✓ 1 tablespoon white sugar
- ✓ 1 1/4 teaspoons salt
- ✓ 1 (1 quart) sterilized canning jar with lid and ring

Directions

1. Process tomatoes, onion, 3 tablespoons and 1/2 teaspoon chopped celery, carrot, beet, green bell pepper, and garlic through a juicer.

2. Stir vegetable juices, water, 1 1/4 teaspoons white sugar, lemon juice, horseradish, Worcestershire sauce, and black pepper together in a large pot. Bring to a boil and cook until flavors blend, about 20 minutes.

3. Sterilize the jars and lids in boiling water for at least 5 minutes. Ladle juice into a quart jar. Stir 1 tablespoon white sugar and 1 teaspoon salt into the juice. Wipe the rim of the jar with a moist paper towel to remove any food residue. Top with lid and screw on ring.

4. Process juice in a pressure canner at 10 pounds of pressure for 35 minutes.

5. Remove the jar from the pressure canner and place onto a cloth-covered or wood surface until cool. Once cool, press the top of the lid with a finger, ensuring that the seal is tight (lid does not move up or down at all). Store in a cool, dark area.

Nutritional Information

- ✓ Calories: 60 kcal 3%
- ✓ Fat: 0.4 g < 1%
- ✓ Carbs: 14.1g 5%
- ✓ Protein: 1.9 g 4%
- ✓ Cholesterol: 0 mg 0%
- ✓ Sodium: 757 mg 30%

Cucumber Orange Carrot Juice

"This is a delicious juice my husband and I make for breakfast or an after-meal dessert when guests are over. It's not only delicious, but will perk up

*any bad day with a boost of vitamins and nutrients that you may
otherwise skip out on. I hope you try it, and enjoy! Recipe makes 2 tall
glasses or 4 smaller glasses of juice. You need a blender."*
Servings: 4 | **Prep**: 10 m | **Ready In**: 10 m

Ingredients

- ✓ 1 large navel orange
- ✓ 2 carrots, roughly chopped
- ✓ 1/2 cucumber, roughly chopped
- ✓ 1/2 cup water, or as needed
- ✓ 1/4 cup white sugar, or to taste
- ✓ 1 teaspoon lemon juice (optional)

Directions

- ✓ Peel orange and save a 1x1-inch piece of the peel. Place orange, orange peel piece, carrots, and cucumber in a blender; pour in water. Blend until desired consistency is reached; add sugar and lemon juice. Blend until smooth, 1 to 3 minutes.

Cook's Note:

- ✓ If you like your juice colder than tap or refrigerated water, add 3 to 6 ice cubes depending on how cold you want your juice.

Nutritional Information

- ✓ Calories: 89 kcal 4%
- ✓ Fat: 0.2 g < 1%
- ✓ Carbs: 22.4g 7%
- ✓ Protein: 0.9 g 2%
- ✓ Cholesterol: 0 mg 0%
- ✓ Sodium: 26 mg 1%

Delicious Green Juice

"An easy, delicious green juice. You can substitute kale for spinach."
***Servings**: 1 | **Prep**: 5 m | **Ready In**: 5 m*

Ingredients

- ✓ 1 cup coconut milk
- ✓ 1 banana
- ✓ 1 mango - peeled, seeded, and chopped
- ✓ 3/4 cup fresh spinach, or to taste

Directions

- ✓ Blend coconut milk, banana, mango, and spinach together in a blender until smooth.

Nutritional Information

- ✓ Calories: 690 kcal 34%
- ✓ Fat: 49.2 g 76%
- ✓ Carbs: 69.3g 22%
- ✓ Protein: 7.6 g 15%
- ✓ Cholesterol: 0 mg 0%
- ✓ Sodium: 52 mg 2%

Drink Your Veggies Pizza

Ingredients

- ✓ 4-5 roma tomatoes
- ✓ 2 bell peppers (yellow, orange)
- ✓ 1/3 yellow onion
- ✓ 1 bunch kale
- ✓ 10-15 basil leaves
- ✓ 1 garlic clove, peeled
- ✓ small handful raw cashew pieces

Directions

- ✓ Juice everything except the cashews. Pour juice into blender with cashews, blend.

Fat Burning Detox Drink

I've got another Detox drink for you! This one is a fat burning concoction that really does the job

Ingredients

- ✓ 12 oz of Water
- ✓ 1-2 Tablespoon Apple Cider Vinegar (I use Braggs with the "Mother")
- ✓ 1 Tablespoon fresh Lemon Juice
- ✓ 1 Teaspoon Cinnamon
- ✓ 1/2 Teaspoon sweetener (I use a Stevia Raw Sugar packet)
- ✓ Half of an apple (sliced)

Directions

1. Put all of the ingredients (not including the Apples) in the blender and blend for about 10 seconds.
2. Add slices of Apple
3. Drink and then eat the apple slices! They will taste yummy.

Festive Cranberry, Pomegranate and Kale Detox Juice

A refreshing, naturally sweet and nourishing juice that combines some key produce of the season, with just a hint of optional mint for an additional festive touch.

Ingredients

- ✓ 4-6 large leaves kale, as you like (add more for more detox properties)

- ✓ 1 cup (240 ml) pomegranate arils (from one large ripe pomegranate)
- ✓ 1 cup (240 ml) fresh or frozen cranberries (if frozen, allow to thaw a bit before juicing)
- ✓ 1 pear, cored
- ✓ one knob (about 1 inch or 2.5 cm) fresh ginger, peeled
- ✓ 6-12 leaves of fresh mint, optional
- ✓ stevia, to taste

Directions

- ✓ Place ingredients in juicer one at a time (I reserved the pomegranate seeds for the end, as their high fiber content pushes out anything else left in the juicer mechanism), strain if desired, and serve immediately. Makes 2 servings.

Ginger Cucumber Apple Detox Juice

Prep: 15 m | Ready In: 15 m

Ingredients

- ✓ Fresh ginger (approx. 3.5 " x 1.5" in size)
- ✓ 1 greenhouse cucumber
- ✓ 3 apples (cored)
- ✓ 1/4 tsp freshly ground allspice
- ✓ Equipment & Utensils
- ✓ Juicer
- ✓ Strainer

Directions

1. Peel ginger and wash cucumber thoroughly.
2. Cut up ginger, cucumber and apples into appropriate sizes to fit into your juicer opening.

3. Juice ginger, cucumber and apples pieces, alternate ingredients when placing into juicer, it helps to push the fruit and veg through more successfully.
4. Once all fruit and veg is juiced, strainer into a jug.
5. To serve, pour juice into glasses and garnish with allspice

Golden Detox Drink

Ingredients

- ✓ 2 cup hot water
- ✓ 2 cups cold water
- ✓ 1/2 tsp turmeric
- ✓ 1/2 small tsp powdered ginger
- ✓ 3 drops Stevia concentrate or 1 tsp raw honey
- ✓ Pinch of cayenne
- ✓ pinch freshly cracked black pepper
- ✓ Juice from 1/2 small organic lemon

Directions

- ✓ Bring 2 cups of water to a boil and while it heats up, put the rest of the ingredients including the 2 cups of cold water in your largest favorite tea cup or jar. Enjoy the drink during the morning or bring any leftovers GDD with you for a boost during the day.

Green Detox Juice

Green detox juice made of cucumber, courgette, pepper, spinach, celeri, apple and ginger cleans your body and supplies it with vitamins and minerals.

Ingredients

- ✓ ½ cucumber

- ✓ ½ courgette
- ✓ Large handful of spinach leafs
- ✓ ½ green bell pepper
- ✓ 2 branches celeri
- ✓ 2 apples
- ✓ 1 cm ginger
- ✓ Juice from ½ lemmon

Directions

- ✓ Wash carefully all the ingredients and peel the ginger. Cut all the veggies and apples into smaller chunks that can enter easily the juicer and throw them in, remember to insert spinach and celeri leafs in between the other large chunks. Collect the juice and add juice from ½ lemmon, mix well with a spoon and serve.

Notes

- ✓ Tip: In order to enjoy better the juice, it is good to use the veggies from the fridge, otherwise you can add few ice cubes.

Green Dragon Veggie Juice

"Energizing and refreshing and a simple way to get your greens! Perfect first thing in the morning or as a savory afternoon treat. I like to add a pinch of salt to really bring out the flavors. I sometimes like to kick it up with a chunk of jalapeno pepper thrown in the mix."

Servings: 1 | **Prep:** 5 m | **Ready In:** 5 m

Ingredients

- ✓ 1/4 large lemon
- ✓ 1 cup fresh spinach, or to taste
- ✓ 2 sprigs fresh parsley, or more to taste
- ✓ 2 stalks celery

- ✓ 1/3 small jalapeno pepper (optional)
- ✓ 1 tomato, quartered
- ✓ 1 pinch salt
- ✓ 1 cup ice, or as desired

Directions

1. Process lemon, spinach, parsley, celery, jalapeno pepper, and tomato, respectively, through a juicer. Season juice with salt.
2. Fill a glass with ice and add juice.

Cook's Note

- ✓ Adjust lemon to your personal preference. If the lemon is small I use half; if larger, I use a quarter or a third. No need to peel the lemon.
- ✓ Since the heat of jalapenos can vary greatly, start out with 1/4 or 1/3 of a small pepper, and adjust accordingly.

Nutritional Information

- ✓ Calories: 74 kcal 4%
- ✓ Fat: 1.1 g 2%
- ✓ Carbs: 16.1g 5%
- ✓ Protein: 4.8 g 10%
- ✓ Cholesterol: 0 mg 0%
- ✓ Sodium: 290 mg 12%

Green Juice

Servings: 1

Ingredients

- ✓ 1/2 head broccoli (or 6 leaves kale), chopped
- ✓ 1 cucumber, chopped
- ✓ 4 stalks celery, chopped

- ✓ 1/4 cup fresh parsley sprigs

Directions

- ✓ Press all ingredients through a juice extractor. Stir and serve immediately.

Green Lemonade

Ingredients

- ✓ 1 apple, cut peel on
- ✓ 1/2 lemon, cut, peel on
- ✓ 1/2-1 head Romaine lettuce, washed
- ✓ 1 large kale leaf or more if desired If using Dino Kale use 2 or more)
- ✓ 1/2 inch ginger, peel on

Directions

- ✓ Juice all ingredients as machine suggests, drink and enjoy.

Heavenly Honeydew Juice

"We had some amazing honeydew juice at a Mexican restaurant and immediately tried to recreate it. We think this is even better than the original!"

Servings: *6* | ***Prep:*** *10 m* | ***Ready In:*** *10 m*

Ingredients

- ✓ 1 (5 pound) honeydew melon, quartered and seeded
- ✓ 2 cups ice cubes
- ✓ 1 cup water
- ✓ 3 tablespoons white sugar

Directions

✓ Scrape flesh from honeydew melon quarters into a blender; add ice cubes, water, and sugar. Blend until smooth and sugar has dissolved. Serve immediately.

Nutritional Information

✓ Calories: 159 kcal 8%

✓ Fat: 0.5 g < 1%

✓ Carbs: 40.3g 13%

✓ Protein: 2 g 4%

✓ Cholesterol: 0 mg 0%

✓ Sodium: 71 mg 3%

Homemade Sports Drink (aka Greaterade)

"The Golden State Warriors' decision to ban commercial sports drinks and make their own with Himalayan sea salt inspired me to try my own-- with less sugar. You can tweak this recipe to create your perfect formula."

Servings: 9 | **Prep**: 10 m | **Cook**: 5 m | **Ready In**: 15 m

Ingredients

✓ 8 cups fresh cold water, divided

✓ 3 tablespoons honey

✓ 1/2 teaspoon fine Himalayan pink salt

✓ 3/4 teaspoon calcium magnesium powder (optional)

✓ 1 pinch cayenne pepper

✓ 3/4 cup freshly squeezed orange juice, strained

✓ 2 lemons, juiced

✓ 2 limes, juiced

Directions

1. Pour 1 cup of the water into a large pot. Add honey, salt, calcium magnesium powder, and cayenne. Place pot over low heat and whisk until ingredients have dissolved.

Remove from heat and allow to return to room temperature.

2. Add juices to room temperature mixture in pot. Pour in remaining 7 cups water and whisk until well blended.

Cook's Note:

✓ This pink salt is NOT the pink salt used to cure meats.

Nutritional Information

✓ Calories: 40 kcal 2%
✓ Fat: 0.1 g < 1%
✓ Carbs: 12.1g 4%
✓ Protein: 0.6 g 1%
✓ Cholesterol: 0 mg 0%
✓ Sodium: 106 mg 4%

Homemade Strawberry Nectar

"They don't sell Strawberry Nectar in my town, so I make my own. The apple juice is for sweetness. Be careful: not all brands have a good aftertaste even frozen. Fresh juiced apple is better. Thawed frozen strawberries may be used when fresh is not available. Be sure to use unsweetened ones."

*Servings: 4 | **Prep**: 10 m | **Ready In**: 10 m*

Ingredients

✓ 2 cups fresh sliced strawberries
✓ 1/4 cup unsweetened apple juice, or to taste
✓ 2 tablespoons water, or as needed (optional)

Directions

✓ Combine the strawberries and apple juice in a blender or food processor. Puree until smooth, then blend in water to your desired thickness.

Nutritional Information

- ✓ Calories: 32 kcal 2%
- ✓ Fat: 0.2 g < 1%
- ✓ Carbs: 7.7g 2%
- ✓ Protein: 0.5 g 1%
- ✓ Cholesterol: 0 mg 0%
- ✓ Sodium: 1 mg < 1%

Homemade Tomato Juice Cocktail

"Delicious tomato juice for a fraction of the cost of store-purchased. Adjust lemon, salt, and sugar to taste. Almost 7 cups of juice for about $1.00! I prefer the natural tomato paste."
***Servings**: 6 | **Prep**: 10 m | **Ready In**: 1 h 10 m*

Ingredients

- ✓ 2 cups water
- ✓ 1 (6 ounce) can tomato paste
- ✓ 2 tablespoons lemon juice
- ✓ 2 tablespoons white sugar
- ✓ 1 teaspoon salt, or to taste
- ✓ 3 cups water, more if needed

Directions

- ✓ Blend 2 cups water, tomato paste, lemon juice, sugar, and salt together in a blender until smooth; pour into a 1/2 gallon container. Stir 3 cups water into mixture. Refrigerate until thickened, about 1 hour. Add 1 more cup water if juice is too thick.

Nutritional Information

- ✓ Calories: 60 kcal 3%
- ✓ Fat: 0.4 g < 1%
- ✓ Carbs: 14.1g 5%

✓ Protein: 1.9 g 4%
✓ Cholesterol: 0 mg 0%
✓ Sodium: 757 mg 30%

Honeydew Agua Fresca

This easy-to-make nonalcoholic drink is inspired by traditional Mexican fruit beverages.

Ingredients

✓ 14 cups honeydew melon or cantaloupe (from a 5-pound melon)
✓ 1/3 cup superfine sugar
✓ 1/2 cup fresh lime juice (from 4 limes)
✓ Ice
✓ 2 cups raspberries

Directions

1. Set a large fine-mesh sieve over a large pitcher or jug. In batches, in a food processor or blender, puree melon until smooth. Pour melon puree through sieve, pressing on solids with a rubber spatula (you should have about 4 cups juice).

2. In a small bowl, combine superfine sugar and fresh lime juice; stir until sugar dissolves. Add lime mixture and 4 cups water to melon juice and mix well. Adjust sweetness with more sugar if desired. (Mixture can be refrigerated, up to 2 days.) To serve, add plenty of ice and 2 cups raspberries.

Honeydew Juice

"A refreshing summer drink. Easier than a piece of cake!"

Servings: 4 | Prep: 10 m | Ready In: 10 m

Ingredients

- ✓ 1 honeydew melon - halved, seeded, and peeled
- ✓ 1 tablespoon honey
- ✓ 1/4 teaspoon white sugar

Directions

- ✓ Blend honeydew, honey, and sugar in a blender on low speed until smooth, about 1 1/2 minutes.

Nutritional Information

- ✓ Calories: 132 kcal 7%
- ✓ Fat: 0.4 g < 1%
- ✓ Carbs: 33.7g 11%
- ✓ Protein: 1.7 g 3%
- ✓ Cholesterol: 0 mg 0%
- ✓ Sodium: 58 mg 2%

Hot Caramel Apple Cider

"Warm up a cold day with a mug of hot apple cider topped with a hint of caramel."

Servings: 4 | Prep: 10 m | Cook: 10 m | Ready In: 20 m

Ingredients

- ✓ 1/4 cup heavy whipping cream
- ✓ 1/4 cup brown sugar
- ✓ 3 cups apple cider
- ✓ 1/2 cup water
- ✓ *Caramel Whipped Cream:*
- ✓ 1/2 cup heavy whipping cream
- ✓ 1 tablespoon brown sugar

Directions

1. Heat 1/4 cup cream and 1/4 cup brown sugar in a saucepan over medium heat until mixture starts to boil. Raise heat to medium-high and stir in apple cider and water. Cook until mixture starts to simmer, about 4 minutes.

2. Beat 1/2 cup cream and 1 tablespoon brown sugar together in a bowl until soft peaks form. Lift your beater or whisk straight up: the whipping cream will form soft mounds rather than a sharp peak.

3. Pour cider into mugs and top with caramel whipped cream.

Cook's Note:

✓ You can substitute apple juice for the cider.

Nutritional Information

✓ Calories: 318 kcal 16%

✓ Fat: 16.5 g 25%

✓ Carbs: 42.9g 14%

✓ Protein: 0.9 g 2%

✓ Cholesterol: 61 mg 20%

✓ Sodium: 43 mg 2%

Hot Carmel Apple Juice

"A great warm fall drink. Great replacement for a winter's hot cocoa! My children love it. I came up with it when I wanted something warm and sweet but didn't want the caffeine. Like hot apple pie in a mug! Top with whipped cream."

Servings: *2* | **Prep:** *5 m* | **Cook:** *5 m* | **Ready In:** *10 m*

Ingredients

✓ 2 cups apple juice

- ✓ 3 tablespoons caramel syrup (such as Hershey's®)
- ✓ 1 teaspoon ground cinnamon
- ✓ 1/2 teaspoon ground nutmeg
- ✓ 1/4 teaspoon vanilla extract
- ✓ 1/4 cup whipped cream, or to taste (optional)

Directions

- ✓ Whisk apple juice, caramel syrup, cinnamon, and nutmeg together in a saucepan over medium-high heat. Cook and whisk briskly until mixture is hot but not boiling, about 3 minutes. Add vanilla; cook and stir for 1 more minute. Pour into mugs and top with whipped cream.

Nutritional Information

- ✓ Calories: 222 kcal 11%
- ✓ Fat: 2.3 g 3%
- ✓ Carbs: 51.5g 17%
- ✓ Protein: 0.9 g 2%
- ✓ Cholesterol: 6 mg 2%
- ✓ Sodium: 125 mg 5%

Lemon Ginger Detox Drink

Ginger is a natural pain reliever and adding it to your water can give you wonderful detox properties.

***Serving**: 1*

Ingredients

- ✓ 1 12-ounce glass water, at room temperature
- ✓ Juice of 1/2 lemon
- ✓ 1/2-inch knob of ginger root

Directions

✓ Add the lemon juice to the glass of water. Finely grate the ginger by using a zester, add to the glass of water. This drink is a perfect way to start your day!

Nutrition Information

✓ Serving Size: 1 drink/full recipe
✓ Calories: 11
✓ Total Fat: 0 g
✓ Saturated Fat: 0 g
✓ Trans Fat: 0 g
✓ Cholesterol: 0 mg
✓ Sodium: 2 mg
✓ Carbohydrates: 0 g
✓ Dietary Fiber: 0 g
✓ Sugars: 1 g
✓ Protein: 0 g
✓ SmartPoints: 0

Love Your Greens Juice

Servings: 1 | Prep: 5 m | Ready In: 5 m

Ingredients

✓ 4 cups baby spinach
✓ ½ head of collards (about 6 leaves)
✓ 1 English cucumber
✓ ½ bunch of parsley (about 1 cup lightly packed)
✓ ½ bunch of cilantro (about ½ cup lightly packed)
✓ Juice from ½ lemon

Directions

- ✓ If you have a 'low' setting on your juicer, juice all items in the recipe but the lemon juice. When complete, add lemon juice, stir and enjoy!

Love Your Liver Juice

Ingredients

- ✓ 2 medium beets
- ✓ 1-inch piece fresh ginger
- ✓ 1 lemon, peeled
- ✓ small handful cilantro
- ✓ 1 chard leaf
- ✓ ½ red apple (optional)

Directions

- ✓ Juice ingredients and enjoy!

Notes

- ✓ Makes one 8 - 12 oz juice

Mango Ginger Lemonade

Ingredients

- ✓ 1/3 cup fresh ginger
- ✓ Juice of 8 meyer lemons
- ✓ 4 champagne mangoes
- ✓ 42 fl oz water
- ✓ 1 1/2 cups agave
- ✓ Ice to serve
- ✓ Blender
- ✓ Skewers

Directions

1. Grate ginger until you have enough to fill 1/3 of a cup.

2. Pour lemon juice into a pitcher and add ginger. Stir and set aside.

3. Slice off one whole side from one of the mangoes and set aside.

4. Extract as much of the flesh of the rest of the mangoes as you can in the most efficient way you can and then place the mango flesh in a blender, top with a couple of tablespoons of water and then blend on the lowest setting on your blender. Leave in blender and set aside.

5. Add water and agave to lemon and ginger and stir.

6. Taste to check intensity of ginger, if you prefer a strong ginger taste, let your ingredients stand for 15-30 mins.

7. Once you have your desired ginger intensity, pour ingredients into blender with mango puree.

8. Blend on lowest setting until ingredients are fully mixed.

9. Slice set aside mango and place on skewers.

10. To serve, pour your mango ginger lemonade over ice and garnish with a mango skewer.

VBLEAN'S ACV Lemon Detox Drink

Ingredients

✓ Cold Water
✓ Ice
✓ Apple Cider Vinegar (With the 'Mother')
✓ Lemon Juice
✓ Optional:
✓ Cinnamon
✓ Stevia

Directions

✓ Mix cold water (I use between 16-25 oz), a few ice cubes, 1-2 tbsp apple cider vinegar (the more you use, the more the detox effect but also the more bitter the drink will be), lemon juice of at least one full lemon, a sprinkle of cinnamon and stevia to taste. Drink entire thing first thing in the morning!

Orange Fizz

"Make boring orange juice tangy and fizzy with this delicious blend!"
***Servings**: 1 | **Prep**: 5 m | **Ready In**: 5 m*

Ingredients
- ✓ ice cubes
- ✓ 1 cup orange juice
- ✓ 1/3 cup tonic water
- ✓ 1 teaspoon lemon juice

Directions
- ✓ Fill a glass with ice cubes. Pour in the orange juice, tonic water and lemon juice. Stir and serve.

Nutritional Information
- ✓ Calories: 140 kcal 7%
- ✓ Fat: 0.5 g < 1%
- ✓ Carbs: 33.2g 11%
- ✓ Protein: 1.8 g 4%
- ✓ Cholesterol: 0 mg 0%
- ✓ Sodium: 19 mg < 1%

Orange Surprise

Ingredients
- ✓ 2 apples, washed and quartered
- ✓ 2 medium carrots, washed, tops removed and cut into large pieces

✓ 1 stalk celery, washed and cut into several pieces
✓ 4-5 calamansi limes, washed

Directions

✓ Process the apples, carrots, celery and lime through a juicer. Serve immediately over ice.

Orange Zinger

"Loaded with vitamins, this is the perfect drink for when you're feeling a little under the weather. The ginger adds a nice, unexpected bite; you can easily adjust ginger quantity to fit your own tastes. This drink is great chilled or served over a few ice cubes."
***Servings**: 1 | **Prep**: 10 m | **Ready In**: 10 m*

Ingredients

✓ 1/2 inch piece fresh ginger root
✓ 1 pound carrots, scrubbed and trimmed
✓ 2 oranges, peeled

Directions

✓ Juice ginger, carrots, and oranges in a juicer, respectively. Serve immediately.

Cook's Note:

✓ Ginger doesn't provide much juice which is why it should go in the juicer first, so that the carrots and oranges can flush the flavor through.

Nutritional Information

✓ Calories: 188 kcal 9%
✓ Fat: 1.1 g 2%
✓ Carbs: 44g 14%
✓ Protein: 4.3 g 9%
✓ Cholesterol: 0 mg 0%
✓ Sodium: 314 mg 13%

Orange, Carrot & Ginger Juice

Ingredients
- ✓ 2 navel oranges peeled
- ✓ 6 large carrots
- ✓ 2 inch piece ginger peeled

Directions
1. Peel oranges and ginger.
2. Cut tops off of carrots.
3. Add ingredients to juicer.
4. Stir and enjoy!

Peach and Mint Juice

"I found out about this from a friend from the Humane Society where I volunteer, just had to share it! If you don't want to wait all night, try using a juicer."

Servings: 5 | Prep: 10 m | Ready In: 8 h 10 m

Ingredients
- ✓ 2 cucumbers, sliced, or more to taste
- ✓ 4 peaches, halved and pitted, or more to taste
- ✓ 2 fresh mint leaves
- ✓ 1 pinch salt

Directions
- ✓ Combine cucumbers, peaches, mint, and salt in a pitcher; stir gently. Refrigerate for 8 hours to overnight.

Cook's Note
- ✓ Experiment! If you don't like peaches, try nectarines or plums.

✓ You can peel the cucumbers if desired. White peaches are preferable.

Nutritional Information

✓ Calories: 37 kcal 2%

✓ Fat: 0.1 g < 1%

✓ Carbs: 8.9g 3%

✓ Protein: 0.8 g 2%

✓ Cholesterol: 0 mg 0%

✓ Sodium: 83 mg 3%

Pineapple Sunrise

"A refreshing way to get your day started with only 3 ingredients but packed full of vitamins! Perfect for those who don't like the overly-sweet flavor of carrot juice. The pineapple and lime really tone down the sweetness."

*Servings: 2 | **Prep**: 10 m | **Ready In**: 10 m*

Ingredients

✓ 1 lime, halved

✓ 1 pound carrots, chopped

✓ 2 cups fresh pineapple chunks

✓ ice, as desired

Directions

✓ Process lime, carrots, and pineapple through a juicer, respectively; serve over ice.

Cook's Notes:

✓ One pound of carrots is about 6 to 7 medium carrots. Once juiced, it makes about 8 ounces of juice.

✓ Two cups fresh pineapple is about 1/3 of a fresh pineapple and makes about 8 ounces of juice. No need to core it.

- ✓ Use only 1/2 the lime if you prefer the juice less tart. No need to peel it.

Nutritional Information

- ✓ Calories: 186 kcal 9%
- ✓ Fat: 0.8 g 1%
- ✓ Carbs: 46.9g 15%
- ✓ Protein: 3.2 g 6%
- ✓ Cholesterol: 0 mg 0%
- ✓ Sodium: 166 mg 7%

Pineapple-Blueberry-Ginger Juice

Blueberries are rich in antioxidants, which have been shown to fight certain types of cancer. The ginger aids digestion, and sets a South Pacific mood when combined with pineapple.
***Servings:** 1 | **Yield:** Makes 10 Ounce*

Ingredients

- ✓ 1/4 pineapple
- ✓ 1 cup blueberries
- ✓ 1 piece fresh ginger (1/4 to 1/2 inch)
- ✓ Juicer

Directions

- ✓ Cut large produce into chunks, and remove big seeds or pits. Don't worry about those in fruits like apples and pears -- the juicer will filter them out. To combine several fruits and vegetables, alternate between soft pieces and hard ones. Finish with the latter to push through anything that's stuck.

Pineapple Spinach Juice

Lettuce juice? Here it's mixed with spinach and pineapple.
***Servings:** 1*

Ingredients

- ✓ 1 cup baby spinach
- ✓ 5 cups chopped romaine
- ✓ 3 cups chopped pineapple

Directions

- ✓ Press spinach, romaine, and pineapple through a juice extractor. Stir and serve immediately.

Polynesian Watermelon Drink ('Otai)

"Otai' is a fruit drink which originated in Tonga and is usually made as a summertime refreshment. It is a blend of water, coconut milk, and any variety of pulped tropical fruit such as coconut, watermelon, mango, and pineapple but is almost always watermelon as it is plentiful in Tonga. A small amount of sugar may be added, although the recipe is considerably sweet on its own. I lived in Sydney many moons ago and the Polynesian families drank this by the gallons in the summer. Soooo refreshing and yummy! Serve over ice cubes."
***Servings:** 12 | **Prep:** 15 m | **Ready In:** 15 m*

Ingredients

- ✓ 1 seedless watermelon, halved and sliced
- ✓ 3 cups water
- ✓ 1 (15.25 ounce) can crushed pineapple
- ✓ 1 (12 fluid ounce) can evaporated milk
- ✓ 1/2 cup shredded coconut
- ✓ 2 tablespoons white sugar, or to taste (optional)
- ✓ 1/2 lime, juiced

Directions

✓ Grate watermelon with a fork from the rind into a large bowl, leaving no large chunks. Stir water, pineapple, evaporated milk, and coconut into the grated watermelon. Add sugar; stir until dissolved. Squeeze lime juice into the watermelon mixture.

Nutritional Information

✓ Calories: 199 kcal
✓ Fat: 3.8 g
✓ Carbs: 41.1g
✓ Protein: 4.7 g
✓ Cholesterol: 9 mg
✓ Sodium: 48 mg

Pomegranate Pineapple Lemon Juice

Ingredients

✓ 1 cup Chopped Pineapple
✓ 1/2 cup Pomegranate juice (I used Pom)
✓ 1 ½ cup Water
✓ Juice of 1/2 lemon
✓ 1 inch piece of Ginger

Directions

1. In a blender combine everything except pomegranate juice and blend together to form a smooth consistency and strain through the strainer and set aside. To Pineapple lemon ginger mixtures mix in Pomegranate juice.

2. Enjoy with ice.

Pomegranate Citrus Juice

Citrus never becomes boring when you mix together juice from a variety of fruits, including grapefruits, oranges, tangerines, and tangelos. Add pomegranate juice for a dose of color, flavor, and antioxidants.
***Servings:** 2*

Ingredients
- ✓ 2 small grapefruits
- ✓ 2 juice oranges
- ✓ 2 tangerines or mineola tangelos
- ✓ 1/2 lime
- ✓ 2 pomegranates

Directions
- ✓ Use a citrus press or a juicer to juice the grapefruits, oranges, tangerines, and lime. Juice the pomegranates (2/3 cup juice) into a separate bowl. Divid citrus juice among 3 glasses. Top with pomegranate juice, which will settle to the bottom, and serve.

Rainbow Veggie Juice

Ingredients
- ✓ 1-2 red bell peppers, seeded and sliced
- ✓ 4 tomatoes, sliced
- ✓ 3 medium carrots, peeled and sliced
- ✓ 2 heads of romaine lettuce
- ✓ 1 bunch of celery
- ✓ large handful of parsley
- ✓ large handful of cilantro
- ✓ 1 English cucumber, peeled and chopped

- ✓ 2 meyer lemons, peeled
- ✓ 1 inch of ginger root

Directions

- ✓ Juice all of your lovely veggies. Give your juice a good stir. Put it in mason jars. Drink it as soon as possible, not waiting longer than 48 hours! Simple, simple.

Raspberry Lemonade

Ingredients

- ✓ 1 cup sugar
- ✓ 1 cup of water
- ✓ ¾ cup raspberries; pureed and pushed through a fine mesh sieve; plus more whole berries for garnish if desired
- ✓ 1 cup fresh lemon juice (this equaled close to 8 of my lemons)
- ✓ 4-6 cups cold water (this will vary depending on your taste)

Directions

1. Make a simple syrup by combining the sugar with 1 cup of water in a saucepan. Place over medium heat and heat until the sugar in completely dissolved; swirl the pan occasionally. Let cool.
2. Measure 3/4 of fresh raspberries and puree them in your blender or food processor.
3. Push the raspberry puree through a fine mesh sieve to separate the seeds from the pulp.
4. Once the simple syrup has cooled, combine the raspberry puree, simple syrup and lemon juice in a large pitcher.

5. Add 4-6 cups of cold water. The amount of water you use will depend on your taste, so add as little or as much as you want to achieve your perfect sweet/tart balance.

Refreshing Tangy Cucumber Juice

"This summertime beauty and health drink is one of my favorite drinks in summer. Drink chilled to get refreshingly cool in the summer. It prevents dehydration in the body."
*Servings: 2 | **Prep**: 10 m | **Ready In**: 10 m*

Ingredients
- ✓ 2 cucumbers, peeled and cut into small pieces
- ✓ 1 cup water, or as needed
- ✓ 1 green chile pepper
- ✓ 6 fresh mint leaves
- ✓ salt to taste
- ✓ 2 teaspoons lime juice

Directions
- ✓ Blend cucumbers, water, green chile pepper, mint, and salt together in a blender until juice is smooth. Pour juice into glasses and add 1 teaspoon lime juice to each glass.

Nutritional Information
- ✓ Calories: 34 kcal 2%
- ✓ Fat: 0.4 g < 1%
- ✓ Carbs: 7.6g 2%
- ✓ Protein: 1.6 g 3%
- ✓ Cholesterol: 0 mg 0%
- ✓ Sodium: 203 mg 8%

Sesame Seed Juice

"A toasted tasty juice, this is a traditional beverage of Puerto Rico. It's so refreshing and a different idea. For an iced cool beverage, add crushed ice and serve immediately."

*Servings: 32 | **Prep**: 10 m | **Cook**: 5 m | **Ready In**: 1 h 15 m*

Ingredients

- ✓ 16 ounces sesame seeds
- ✓ 2 cups white sugar
- ✓ 1 gallon water, or as needed

Directions

1. Cook sesame seeds in a large saucepan over medium heat, stirring constantly, until seeds are toasted and fragrant, about 5 minutes. Remove saucepan from heat and cover with a lid.
2. Place sugar in a blender and pour in enough water to fill halfway; add seeds. Blend sugar-seed mixture until smooth; pour through a fine-mesh strainer into a pitcher. Repeat blending and straining if a thinner drink is desired, adding more water as desired. Refrigerate juice until cooled, about 1 hour.

Nutritional Information

- ✓ Calories: 129 kcal 6%
- ✓ Fat: 7 g 11%
- ✓ Carbs: 15.8g 5%
- ✓ Protein: 2.5 g 5%
- ✓ Cholesterol: 0 mg 0%
- ✓ Sodium: 5 mg < 1%

Shikaji – India Masala Lemonade

Ingredients

- ✓ 1 big lemon

- ✓ Chilled water - 2 glasses
- ✓ Rock Salt/sendha namak – ¼ tsp
- ✓ Black pepper – ¼ tsp
- ✓ Roasted Cumin seeds - ¼ tsp (crushed)
- ✓ Sugar – 4 tsp
- ✓ Few Mint leaves and Lemon Slices to garnish
- ✓ Ice cubes – 6-8

Directions

1. Divide lemon into equal half. Microwave it for 10 seconds. Squeeze it nicely to take out the maximum juice.
2. Add water, lemon juice, sugar, rock salt, black pepper, roasted cumin seeds in a jar and mix well.
3. Pour it in a serving glass with ice-cubes and garnish lemon slices and mint leaves.

Skinny Detox Juice

Here is the most complete detox agent in the world; however, there is one caveat. This one is not necessarily water. Unlike all of the other entries on this list, the last slot is occupied by a bona fide juice.

Ingredients

- ✓ 2 pears (cored)
- ✓ 2 carrots
- ✓ 2 stalks celery
- ✓ 2 nectarines (pits removed)
- ✓ 1 lemon (remove the rind leaving most of the white on)
- ✓ 2 cups honeydew melon cubed
- ✓ 1 orange (remove rind leaving most of the white on)
- ✓ 1 inch piece ginger

Directions

- ✓ Juice all the ingredients in the order they are listed. If you want to add some greens, feel free. I have not been able to get my daughter to drink the green juice yet. I will keep trying though! Try to drink your juice within the first 12-24 hours to get the most benefits. If you go longer, some of the enzymes may be lost. I got about 25oz of juice out of this recipe. Enjoy!

Sour Berry Blast Slushy

"I love making this recipe for my friends, family, and just for myself! I love the sour kick. It's funny if you don't tell the person who you served it to that it's sour! Great for parties, summer, and get-togethers."
*Servings: 2 | **Prep**: 5 m | **Ready In**: 5 m*

Ingredients

- ✓ 8 ice cubes
- ✓ 3/4 cup water
- ✓ 1/2 cup frozen mixed berries
- ✓ 1/2 cup fresh mixed berries
- ✓ 1/4 cup lemon juice, or to taste
- ✓ 2 tablespoons white sugar (optional)
- ✓ 1 splash orange juice (optional)

Directions

- ✓ Blend ice cubes, water, frozen berries, fresh berries, lemon juice, sugar, and orange juice together in a blender until a slushy consistency is reached, about 30 seconds.

Cook's Note

- ✓ To make recipe less tart, add more sugar or less lemon juice.

✓ More ice cubes will make slushy less like juice and more like something you would eat with a spoon.

Nutritional Information

Calories: 105 kcal 5%

Fat: 0.2 g < 1%

Carbs: 27.1g 9%

Protein: 0.9 g 2%

Cholesterol: 0 mg 0%

Sodium: 7 mg < 1%

Soursop Punch

"One of my favorite beverages when I was a little girl was made with the soursop fruit. You can use either white or brown sugar for this punch."
***Servings**: 1 | **Prep**: 15 m | **Ready In**: 45 m*

Ingredients

✓ 1 soursop fruit, peeled and cut into chunks

✓ 1 1/2 cups milk, or to taste

✓ 2 tablespoons white sugar, or to taste

✓ 2 teaspoons vanilla extract

✓ 1/2 teaspoon ground cinnamon

✓ 1/4 teaspoon ground nutmeg

Directions

1. Working in batches, press soursop pieces through a fine-mesh strainer with the back of a spoon into a bowl to remove the juice from the fruit.
2. Whisk milk, sugar, vanilla, cinnamon, and nutmeg into soursop juice until sugar is dissolved completely. Pour punch into a pitcher and refrigerate until chilled, at least 30 minutes.

Nutritional Information

- ✓ Calories: 724 kcal 36%
- ✓ Fat: 9.4 g 14%
- ✓ Carbs: 149.8g 48%
- ✓ Protein: 18.4 g 37%
- ✓ Cholesterol: 29 mg 10%
- ✓ Sodium: 239 mg 10%

Spicy Tomato Drink

"Very tasty drink, high in potassium. Not just bland tomato juice. Serve as is or add vodka for the best Bloody Mary."
Servings: 6 | **Prep**: 5 m | **Ready In**: 1 h 5 m

Ingredients

- ✓ 1 (46 fluid ounce) can tomato juice
- ✓ 1/2 cup cider vinegar
- ✓ 1/3 cup white sugar
- ✓ 3 tablespoons prepared horseradish
- ✓ 2 tablespoons Worcestershire sauce
- ✓ 2 tablespoons adobo seasoning
- ✓ 1 tablespoon onion powder

Directions

- ✓ Combine tomato juice, vinegar, sugar, horseradish, Worcestershire sauce, adobo seasoning, and onion powder in a 2-quart container. Mix well and chill for at least 1 hour.

Nutritional Information

- ✓ Calories: 102 kcal 5%
- ✓ Fat: 0.5 g < 1%
- ✓ Carbs: 24.4g 8%
- ✓ Protein: 2.1 g 4%

✓ Cholesterol: 0 mg 0%
✓ Sodium: 659 mg 26%

Spicy Tomato Juice

When you want a Bloody Mary kick, but can do without the vodka.

Ingredients

✓ 3 stalks of celery, leaves attached
✓ 1 cup chopped tomatoes
✓ 1 jalapeno, seeded and minced
✓ 1/4 cup freshly squeezed lemon juice
✓ 1/8 teaspoon celery seed
✓ 1/8 teaspoon freshly ground pepper
✓ 1/4 teaspoon coarse salt
✓ 2 red chile peppers, for garnish (optional)

Directions

1. Place celery in a juice extractor; process, extracting about 1/2 cup juice. Transfer to bowl of a food processor or jar of a blender.
2. Add chopped tomatoes, jalapeno, lemon juice, celery seed, black pepper, and salt. Process until fairly smooth, with some texture remaining. Garnish with chile peppers, and serve over ice, if desired.

Spinach CucumberCelery Juice

Because celery isn't overpowering, it allows the spinach and cucumber juices to stand out. Spinach is a good source of calcium, iron, and potassium.

Serving: 1

Ingredients

- ✓ 2 cups packed spinach (4 ounces)
- ✓ 1 cucumber
- ✓ 1 celery stalk
- ✓ Juicer

Directions

- ✓ Cut large produce into chunks, and remove big seeds or pits. Don't worry about those in fruits like apples and pears -- the juicer will filter them out. To combine several fruits and vegetables, alternate between soft pieces and hard ones. Finish with the latter to push through anything that's stuck.

Strawberry Mint Chia Fresca

"Refreshing, healthy, and energizing drink containing coconut water for electrolytes and mint for a cool taste. Chia seeds are high in omega-3 fatty acids and antioxidants. Inspired by Mexican Chia Fresca and my love for mojitos! The juice can be drunk without waiting the 30 minutes, but the seeds might stick to the glass more. A juicer can be used to juice the strawberries and mint. Doing so will give more mint flavor and may require using less mint to begin with."
Servings: 8 | **Prep**: 15 m | **Ready In**: 15 m

Ingredients

- ✓ 2 cups ripe strawberries
- ✓ 1 cup water
- ✓ 1 cup fresh mint leaves
- ✓ 2 (17.5 ounce) cans coconut
- ✓ water water
- ✓ 1/4 cup lime juice
- ✓ 1/4 cup lemon juice

- ✓ 2 tablespoons agave nectar
- ✓ 1/3 cup chia seeds

Directions

1. Blend strawberries, 1 cup water, and mint leaves in a blender until smooth, 20 to 30 seconds; strain into a 2-quart pitcher. Stir coconut water, 1 cup water, lime juice, lemon juice, and agave nectar into the strawberry mixture.

2. Mix chia seeds in small increments into the strawberry mixture, stirring continually to keep from clumping together. Refrigerate mixture until chia seeds fully absorb the liquid, 30 minutes to overnight.

Nutritional Information

- ✓ Calories: 82 kcal 4%
- ✓ Fat: 1.9 g 3%
- ✓ Carbs: 15.5g 5%
- ✓ Protein: 2.1 g 4%
- ✓ Cholesterol: 0 mg 0%
- ✓ Sodium: 141 mg 6%

Sugar Free Indian Gooseberry Drink

Ingredients

- ✓ Amla (Gooseberry/Nellikka) – 7 or 8 medium to large size
- ✓ Lemon zest- ½ tspn
- ✓ Lemon- ½ sliced into thin slices
- ✓ Mint leaves- 2 sprigs
- ✓ Cold water- 7 cups
- ✓ Salt- 1 tbsp(or to taste)

Directions

1. Discard the seeds of Amla.

2. Dump in the flesh of Amla, lemon zest, salt and water into you mixer aka juicer.
3. Strain the juice.
4. Crush the mint leaves between you palm and add it with lemon pieces to the juice.
5. Serve chilled and get healthy

Summer Watermelon Detox Juice

When your body is begging for hydration, smaller portions, and fresh or even raw foods, turn to this refreshing summer detox juice recipe.

Ingredients

- ✓ 4 cups watermelon chunks, chilled
- ✓ 4-5 romaine lettuce leaves
- ✓ 1 lime, freshly squeezed
- ✓ 1/2" fresh ginger, peeled (optional)
- ✓ 1 tablespoon fresh-chopped mint (optional)
- ✓ 1/2" piece jalapeno (optional)
- ✓ 2 teaspoons honey
- ✓ 1 tablespoon coarse sea salt

Directions

1. Place watermelon, romaine, lime juice, ginger, mint, and jalapeno (if desired) in a blender. Blend until pureed.
2. Rim two glasses with honey, dip in salt. Pour juice into prepared glasses. Sip immediately and enjoy.

Notes

- ✓ If making for breakfast, be sure to include 2 Tbsp of hemp seeds to bump up the protein!

Super Green Detox Drink

This Super Green Detox Drink is the perfect beverage to whip up after a night of indulging.

***Serving**: 1*

Ingredients

- ✓ 2 celery stalks, chopped
- ✓ 1 small cucumber, chopped
- ✓ 2 kale leaves
- ✓ 1 handful spinach
- ✓ Handful of fresh parsley or cilantro
- ✓ 1 lemon peeled
- ✓ 1 apple, seeded, cored and chopped

Directions

1. If using a juicer: Add all the above ingredients to a juicer and juice.

2. If using a high powered blender: Add all the above ingredients to a blender along with 1 cup chilled water. Add ice if desired. Blend until smooth. If no pulp is desired, strain smoothie through a fine mesh strainer before drinking.

Super Hydration Juice

Ingredients

- ✓ 2-3 organic cucumbers, large
- ✓ 2 organic apples
- ✓ 1/4 organic beet or a handful of organic strawberries (opt)*
- ✓ Organic mint, to taste

Directions

- ✓ Juice everything together in your juicer. Pour into two glasses with ice. Add a couple sprigs of mint for a garnish. Enjoy!

Super Veggie Juice With A Kick

"A healthy and flavorful fresh juice to help you load up on those servings of veggies that may otherwise be difficult to consume. Add some ginger for a little kick. It's better if they're all chilled before juicing or shake the juice in a cocktail shaker with some ice just to chill, then strain the ice out before drinking."

*Servings: 1 | **Prep**: 10 m | **Ready In**: 10 m*

Ingredients

- ✓ 2 large carrots, ends trimmed
- ✓ 2 large celery stalks
- ✓ 1/2 beet
- ✓ 1/4 green bell pepper
- ✓ 1/4 apple
- ✓ 1/2 teaspoon chopped fresh ginger (optional)

Directions

- ✓ Run carrots, celery, beet, green bell pepper, apple, and ginger through a juicer according to manufacturer's instructions.

Nutritional Information

- ✓ Calories: 122 kcal 6%
- ✓ Fat: 0.7 g 1%
- ✓ Carbs: 27.8g 9%
- ✓ Protein: 3.2 g 6%
- ✓ Cholesterol: 0 mg 0%
- ✓ Sodium: 235 mg 9%

Tamarind Agua Fresca

"This is another favorite agua fresca drink of mine. The tamarind has a sweet and sour kind of taste to it. You can find tamarind concentrate in most Mexican or Asian markets. Serve immediately or chill until ready to serve."

Servings: *4* | ***Prep***: *10 m* | ***Ready In***: *10 m*

Ingredients

- ✓ ice
- ✓ 6 cups water
- ✓ 1/3 cup tamarind concentrate
- ✓ 1/3 cup white sugar
- ✓ 1 orange, thinly sliced
- ✓ 1 lime, thinly sliced

Directions

- ✓ Fill glasses with ice. Combine water, tamarind concentrate, and sugar in a pitcher; stir until sugar is dissolved. Pour over ice and garnish with orange and lime slices.

Nutritional Information

- ✓ Calories: 84 kcal 4%
- ✓ Fat: 0.1 g < 1%
- ✓ Carbs: 21.7g 7%
- ✓ Protein: 0.4 g < 1%
- ✓ Cholesterol: 0 mg 0%
- ✓ Sodium: 13 mg < 1%

Thanksgiving Refreshment

"Sparkling juice beverage."

Servings: 1 | Prep: 5 m | Ready In: 5 m

Ingredients

- ✓ 2 cups vanilla soy milk
- ✓ 1 cup fresh pineapple chunks
- ✓ 2/3 cup frozen cantaloupe chunks
- ✓ 1/2 cup soft tofu
- ✓ 2 tablespoons lime juice
- ✓ 1 1/2 teaspoons coconut extract

Directions

- ✓ Fill a tall glass with ice; add cranberry juice and top with sparkling water. Garnish drink with a lime wedge.

Cook's Note:

- ✓ Frozen banana chunks sub well in place of the cantaloupe.

Nutritional Information

- ✓ Calories: 138 kcal 7%
- ✓ Fat: 0.3 g < 1%
- ✓ Carbs: 34.7g 11%
- ✓ Protein: 0 g < 1%
- ✓ Cholesterol: 0 mg 0%
- ✓ Sodium: 11 mg < 1%

The Apple Cider Soda Detox Beverage

Trying to detox from a soda habit? Mix up this refreshing, all-natural bubbly and sip your way to soda free.

Prep: 1 m

Ingredients

- ✓ 1 1/2 tablespoons organic apple cider vinegar
- ✓ 16 ounces sparkling mineral water

- ✓ juice of 1 lemon
- ✓ stevia to taste
- ✓ ice

Directions

- ✓ Mix all ingredients together over ice. Add just a drop or two of stevia if desired--just enough to slightly sweeten the drink.

Notes

1. For the first 2 weeks, enjoy this drink 2-3 times daily.
2. After that, enjoy it once daily. Preferably drinking it 20 minutes before eating.

The Apple Cider Soda Detox Beverage

This simple ginger punch is the hottest health craze since kombucha. A simple way to increase your daily intake of alkalizing apple cider vinegar, this delicious drink is also an ideal way to kick a soda habit.

***Prep**: 1 m | **Ready In**: 2 h 5 m*

Ingredients

- ✓ 1 1/2 tablespoons organic apple cider vinegar
- ✓ 16 ounces sparkling mineral water
- ✓ juice of 1 lemon
- ✓ stevia to taste
- ✓ ice

Directions

- ✓ Place all ingredients in a 1 quart mason jar. Cover and refrigerate for at least 2 hours. Shake before drinking (you may also want to strain the mixture through a fine-mesh strain to remove the ginger). If desired, serve over ice or mix with soda water. Garnish with fresh mint, if desired.

Triple Fruit Drink

"Great drink for brunch. Great mixture of orange, lemon, and apricot nectar."
***Servings**: 4 | **Prep**: 5 m | **Ready In**: 5 m*

Ingredients

- ✓ 1 (12 ounce) can apricot nectar, chilled
- ✓ 1 1/2 cups orange juice, chilled
- ✓ 2 tablespoons lemon juice

Directions

- ✓ In a pitcher, combine apricot nectar, orange juice, and lemon juice. Serve chilled.

Nutritional Information

- ✓ Calories: 91 kcal 5%
- ✓ Fat: 0.3 g < 1%
- ✓ Carbs: 22.6g 7%
- ✓ Protein: 1 g 2%
- ✓ Cholesterol: 0 mg 0%
- ✓ Sodium: 4 mg < 1%

Tropical Teaser Smoothie

"This non-dairy smoothie was created on a cold snowy day so that I could imagine that I was on a tropical beach somewhere. Lime juice and coconut extract give it a colada taste."
***Servings**: 2 | **Prep**: 10 m | **Ready In**: 10 m*

Ingredients

- ✓ 2 cups vanilla soy milk
- ✓ 1 cup fresh pineapple chunks

- ✓ 2/3 cup frozen cantaloupe chunks
- ✓ 1/2 cup soft tofu
- ✓ 2 tablespoons lime juice
- ✓ 1 1/2 teaspoons coconut extract

Directions

- ✓ Blend soy milk, pineapple, cantaloupe, tofu, lime juice, and coconut extract in a blender until smooth.

Cook's Note

- ✓ Frozen banana chunks sub well in place of the cantaloupe.

Nutritional Information

- ✓ Calories: 230 kcal 12%
- ✓ Fat: 6.9 g 11%
- ✓ Carbs: 29.9g 10%
- ✓ Protein: 12.5 g 25%
- ✓ Cholesterol: 0 mg 0%
- ✓ Sodium: 122 mg 5%

Turmeric Ginger C Boost Life Juice

"The medicinal properties of this spice have been slowly revealing themselves over the centuries. Long known for its anti-inflammatory properties, recent research has revealed that turmeric is a natural wonder, proving beneficial in the treatment of many different health conditions."

Servings: *1 |* **Prep:** *5 m |* **Ready In:** *5 m*

Ingredients

- ✓ 2 Fuji apples, cored and sliced
- ✓ 1 orange, peeled and sectioned
- ✓ 1/2 lemon, peeled
- ✓ 1 (1 inch) piece fresh ginger

✓ 1/2 teaspoon ground turmeric

Directions

✓ Process apples, orange, lemon, and ginger through a juicer; stir in turmeric until evenly incorporated.

Editor's Note

✓ Nutrition data for this recipe includes the full amount of fiber. The actual amount of fiber consumed will vary.

Nutritional Information

✓ Calories: 163 kcal 8%

✓ Fat: 0.8 g 1%

✓ Carbs: 45.8g 15%

✓ Protein: 1.6 g 3%

✓ Cholesterol: 0 mg 0%

✓ Sodium: 6 mg < 1%

Ultra Green Juice

"Green juice" is typically a hodgepodge of seasonal green veggies and fruits. Here, the sweetness comes from apple and honeydew.
***Servings**: 2 | **Yield**: Makes 2 1/2 Cups*

Ingredients

✓ 1 bunch kale

✓ 1 Granny Smith apple, cored and quartered

✓ 1 head fennel, quartered

✓ 1-inch piece fresh ginger, peeled

✓ 1 stalk celery

✓ 1/4 honeydew melon, rind and seeds removed

Directions

✓ Press all ingredients through a juice extractor in batches. Stir and serve immediately.

V3 (Tomato, Cucumber, and Pepper Juice)

Our fresh take on the supermarket standard requires only a quick whirl in the blender. It's frothy and delicious -- and surprisingly filling, thanks in part to the vegetables' fibrous pulp.
Servings*: 4*

Ingredients

- ✓ 2 large tomatoes, cored and chopped
- ✓ 1/2 English cucumber, peeled and chopped
- ✓ 1/2 red bell pepper, seeded and chopped
- ✓ 1 small clove garlic, chopped
- ✓ 1 tablespoon lemon juice, plus wedges for serving
- ✓ Coarse salt

Directions

1. Puree ingredients in a blender until smooth.
2. Season with salt and serve with lemon wedges.

V9 Juice

"A tasty veggie beverage. You can also use it for a great soup base."
Servings*: 56 |* ***Prep****: 1 h 30 m |* ***Cook****: 15 m |* ***Ready In****: 9 h 45 m*

Ingredients

- ✓ 27 pounds tomatoes, cored
- ✓ 9 carrots
- ✓ 2 cups green peas
- ✓ 3 large onions
- ✓ 1/2 head cabbage
- ✓ 3 cups fresh spinach
- ✓ 1 green bell pepper
- ✓ 1 red bell pepper

- ✓ 2 1/2 cups broccoli florets
- ✓ 1 acorn squash - halved, seeded, and cut into chunks
- ✓ 1 bunch celery, ribs separated
- ✓ 5 cloves garlic, peeled
- ✓ 1/2 cup lemon juice
- ✓ 1/4 cup sea salt
- ✓ 1 tablespoon ground black pepper
- ✓ 14 1-quart canning jars with lids and rings

Directions

1. Cook tomatoes in a large stock pot over medium heat until tender, about 20 minutes.

2. Juice carrots, peas, onions, cabbage, spinach, red and green bell peppers, broccoli, acorn squash, celery, and garlic in a vegetable juicer according to the manufacturer's instructions. Stir the juice and vegetable pulp into the tomatoes and bring mixture to a boil. Mix in lemon juice, sea salt, and black pepper, stirring to dissolve salt. Process the mixture through a food mill to strain out all seeds, skins, and pulp.

3. Sterilize the jars and lids in boiling water for at least 5 minutes. Pack the vegetable juice into the hot, sterilized jars, filling the jars to within 1/4 inch of the top. Run a knife or a thin spatula around the insides of the jars after they have been filled to remove any air bubbles. Wipe the rims of the jars with a moist paper towel to remove any food residue. Top with lids, and screw on rings.

4. Place a rack in the bottom of a large stockpot and fill halfway with water. Bring to a boil and lower jars into the boiling water using a holder. Leave a 2-inch space between the jars. Pour in more boiling water if necessary to bring the water level to at least 1 inch above the tops

of the jars. Bring the water to a rolling boil, cover the pot, and process for 15 minutes.

5. Remove the jars from the stockpot and place onto a cloth-covered or wood surface, several inches apart, until cool. Once cool, press the top of each lid with a finger, ensuring that the seal is tight (lid does not move up or down at all). Store in a cool, dark area.

Nutritional Information

- ✓ Calories: 63 kcal 3%
- ✓ Fat: 0.6 g < 1%
- ✓ Carbs: 13.7g 4%
- ✓ Protein: 2.9 g 6%
- ✓ Cholesterol: 0 mg 0%
- ✓ Sodium: 414 mg 17%

Vegetable and Fruit Juice

"This is so delicious and addictive! It is also very healthy. It tastes very fresh with the lime and ginger kick at the end of the drink. If you want to save the pulp, juice the carrots and tomatoes in the beginning and then remove the pulp to save for soup. You can add broth and onions and garlic to the pulp and it makes a very tasty soup in minutes!"

Servings: 2 | Prep: 10 m | Ready In: 10 m

Ingredients

- ✓ 3 large carrots
- ✓ 1 large tomato
- ✓ 8 large strawberries
- ✓ 1 lime, sliced
- ✓ 1 (1 inch) piece fresh ginger
- ✓ 1 apple
- ✓ 1 large red bell pepper, stemmed and seeded

Directions

- ✓ Juice carrots, tomato, strawberries, lime slices, ginger, apple, and red bell pepper using a juicer following manufacturer's instructions.

Nutritional Information

- ✓ Calories: 157 kcal 8%
- ✓ Fat: 1.1 g 2%
- ✓ Carbs: 37.9g 12%
- ✓ Protein: 3.6 g 7%
- ✓ Cholesterol: 0 mg 0%
- ✓ Sodium: 85 mg 3%

Vegetable Juice

Veggie juice is rich in vitamins, with less salt than store-bought. You will need an electric juicer for this recipe.

Servings: 2

Ingredients

- ✓ 3 medium (about 1 1/2 pounds) tomatoes, cut into large chunks
- ✓ 7 celery stalks, each cut into 3-inch pieces
- ✓ 1/2 pound carrots, each cut into 3-inch pieces (do not peel)
- ✓ 1 piece fresh horseradish, (2 1/2 by 1/4 inches), peeled (or 2 1/2 teaspoons prepared horseradish)
- ✓ 1/4 teaspoon coarse salt
- ✓ 2 1/2 teaspoons freshly squeezed lemon juice, plus lemon wedges, for serving

Directions

- ✓ Working in batches, press the tomatoes, celery, carrots, and horseradish through an electric juicer into a large bowl. Stir in salt and lemon juice. Pour vegetable mixture through a fine sieve into another large bowl or a pitcher. Divide vegetable juice evenly between 2 glasses. Serve each with a lemon wedge.

V-Great Juice

"This is the first juice I made, and I hit it out of the ballpark by just using what I had on hand."
Servings: 1 | Prep: 15 m | Ready In: 15 m

Ingredients
- ✓ 4 tomatoes (such is Kumato®)
- ✓ 4 carrots
- ✓ 4 stalks celery
- ✓ 1/2 cup mixed spring greens, or to taste
- ✓ 2 leaves kale
- ✓ 3 radishes
- ✓ 1/4 lemon, with rind
- ✓ 1/4 lemon, peeled

Directions
- ✓ Run tomatoes, carrots, celery, spring greens, kale, radishes, lemon with rind, and peeled lemon through a juicer according to manufacturer's instructions.

Cook's Note
1. I used a Breville Juice Fountain Plus(R) to make this; I used low speed for everything except the carrots and radishes.
2. Don't forget to add a liner or bag to the refuse bin if your juicer model has that feature.

Nutritional Information
- ✓ Calories: 288 kcal 14%

- ✓ Fat: 2.7 g 4%
- ✓ Carbs: 66.8g 22%
- ✓ Protein: 11.5 g 23%
- ✓ Cholesterol: 0 mg 0%
- ✓ Sodium: 387 mg 15%

Virgin Sunset

"This is my interpretation of a virgin sunset. I also refer to this as a pineapple, orange, cherry cocktail. The grenadine will sink to bottom causing layering of orange and red, hence, 'sunset.' If you wanted to make this alcoholic, a shot of champagne is my favorite, but tequila and vodka are other good alternatives. Flavored schnapps may also be an interesting mix."

Servings: 1 | Prep: 5 m | Ready In: 5 m

Ingredients

- ✓ Ice cubes
- ✓ 1/4 cup orange juice
- ✓ 1/4 cup pineapple juice
- ✓ 1/4 cup cranberry juice
- ✓ 1 splash grenadine syrup

Directions

- ✓ Fill a glass with ice. Pour orange juice, pineapple juice, and cranberry juice over the ice and stir. Float a splash of grenadine syrup atop the mixture and serve.

Nutritional Information

- ✓ Calories: 161 kcal 8%
- ✓ Fat: 0.3 g < 1%
- ✓ Carbs: 39.5g 13%
- ✓ Protein: 0.7 g 1%
- ✓ Cholesterol: 0 mg 0%

✓ Sodium: 12 mg < 1%

Watermelon and Bell Pepper Slush

"Light, refreshing, and super simple. It's naturally sweet and a perfect treat for a summer day. Actually, they sell the same exact thing in a tourist town in Florida for $5 a glass! Use sweet red, orange, or yellow bell peppers."
*Servings: 4 | **Prep**: 10 m | **Ready In**: 10 m*

Ingredients
✓ 3 cups cubed seeded watermelon
✓ 1/2 red bell pepper, seeded and coarsely chopped
✓ 3 cups ice
✓ 1 sprig fresh mint

Directions
✓ Place the watermelon, red bell pepper, and ice in a blender, and blend until the ice is crushed and the drink is slushy. Pour into glasses, and garnish with fresh mint leaves. Can be stored in refrigerator up to 2 days.

Cook's Note:
✓ Do not use green bell pepper, because it tends to be more bitter than the red or yellow peppers.

Nutritional Information
✓ Calories: 40 kcal 2%
✓ Fat: 0.2 g < 1%
✓ Carbs: 9.7g 3%
✓ Protein: 0.9 g 2%
✓ Cholesterol: 0 mg 0%
✓ Sodium: 7 mg < 1%

Watermelon Cooler

"Refreshing and healthy! Works best served with big straws! Feel free to leave some big chunks."
*Servings: 8 | **Prep**: 15 m | **Ready In**: 15 m*

Ingredients
- ✓ 1 small watermelon, seeded and cubed

Directions
- ✓ Blend watermelon cubes in a blender until smooth. Chill before serving.

Nutritional Information
- ✓ Calories: 51 kcal 3%
- ✓ Fat: 0.3 g < 1%
- ✓ Carbs: 12.9g 4%
- ✓ Protein: 1 g 2%
- ✓ Cholesterol: 0 mg 0%
- ✓ Sodium: 2 mg < 1%

Watermelon Juice

"A quick and delicious drink that goes well on any day. You can even make ice pops out of this drink as a snack. Try lemon-lime soda in place of water for another variation. You can also add ice cubes if you want it colder and somewhat slushy."
*Servings: 4 | **Prep**: 4 m | **Ready In**: 5 m*

Ingredients
- ✓ 2 cups diced seedless watermelon
- ✓ 2 cups water
- ✓ 1 tablespoon white sugar, or more to taste (optional)

Directions

- ✓ Blend watermelon, water, and sugar in a blender until smooth.

Nutritional Information

- ✓ Calories: 35 kcal 2%
- ✓ Fat: 0.1 g < 1%
- ✓ Carbs: 8.9g 3%
- ✓ Protein: 0.5 g < 1%
- ✓ Cholesterol: 0 mg 0%
- ✓ Sodium: 4 mg < 1%

Watermelon Lime Agua Fresca

"A very refreshing drink. You may also use cantaloupe or honeydew melon. These taste like the juices served in authentic Mexican restaurants. Serve in tall glasses over ice."

Servings: 10 | **Prep**: 15 m | **Ready In**: 1 h 15 m

Ingredients

- ✓ 8 cups water, divided
- ✓ 5 cups peeled, cubed, and seeded watermelon
- ✓ 1/2 cup white sugar, or more to taste
- ✓ 1/3 cup lime juice, or more to taste

Directions

- ✓ Combine 1 cup water, watermelon, and sugar in a blender; process until smooth. Pour into a large pitcher; stir in lime juice and remaining 7 cups water. Taste; adjust sugar or lime juice. Refrigerate until chilled, about 1 hour.

Nutritional Information

- ✓ Calories: 64 kcal 3%
- ✓ Fat: 0.1 g < 1%

✓ Carbs: 16.4g 5%
✓ Protein: 0.5 g < 1%
✓ Cholesterol: 0 mg 0%
✓ Sodium: 7 mg < 1%
✓

Watermelon Summertime Slush

"A crisp and refreshing summertime treat! This drink is a great afternoon pick-me-up."

Servings: *2* | ***Prep***: *10 m* | ***Ready In***: *10 m*

Ingredients

✓ 1 cup ice cubes
✓ 1/2 cup coconut water (liquid from inside coconut)
✓ 1/4 cup cherries, pitted
✓ 1 cup cubed, seeded watermelon
✓ 1 teaspoon granular sucralose sweetener (such as Splenda®) (optional)

Directions

✓ Place ice in a blender and pour in coconut water; add cherries, watermelon cubes, and sweetener. Cover and blend until slushy, about 1 minute. Pour into 2 glasses to serve.

Cook's Note

✓ A variety of fruit can be added to this recipe such as blueberries, strawberries, melon, etc. Blackberries and raspberries are not recommended because of the seeds. A variety of sweeteners can be used for this recipe, or none at all. Some possibilities would be cane sugar, honey, Splenda(R), or agave.

Nutritional Information

✓ Calories: 49 kcal 2%

- ✓ Fat: 0.4 g < 1%
- ✓ Carbs: 11.7g 4%
- ✓ Protein: 1.1 g 2%
- ✓ Cholesterol: 0 mg 0%
- ✓ Sodium: 67 mg 3%

Whole Food Spicy Green "Juice"

Ingredients

- ✓ 2 big handfuls of spinach
- ✓ About 1/4 cup parsley
- ✓ 1 stalk celery, cut into chunks
- ✓ 1 small cucumber, peeled
- ✓ 1 inch piece of ginger, peeled
- ✓ Juice of 1 lemon
- ✓ 6 ice cubes plus enough water to blend

Directions

1. Place all ingredients into a high-powered blender. Blend until everything is smooth and frothy.
2. Drink immediately, as this "juice" will separate.

Yummy Mango Citrus Drink

"This is a modified version of one of the expensive all natural drinks sold commercially! Enjoy!"
Servings: 2 | Prep: 10 m | Ready In: 10 m

Ingredients

- ✓ 1 banana, peeled
- ✓ 1/2 lemon, peeled
- ✓ 1 mango - peeled, seeded, and cut into wedges
- ✓ 1/2 orange, peeled

- ✓ 2 apples, cut into chunks
- ✓ 2 slices fresh ginger root

Directions

- ✓ Process banana, lemon, mango, orange, apples, and ginger through juicer.

Nutritional Information

- ✓ Calories: 180 kcal 9%
- ✓ Fat: 0.7 g 1%
- ✓ Carbs: 48.5g 16%
- ✓ Protein: 1.7 g 3%
- ✓ Cholesterol: 0 mg 0%
- ✓ Sodium: 5 mg < 1%

Three: Detox Smoothie

***

Antioxidant Smoothie

Unsweetened pomegranate juice blended with mixed berries makes a refreshing frozen drink.
Servings: 2

Ingredients

- ✓ 2 cups mixed frozen berries (9 ounces)
- ✓ 1 cup unsweetened pomegranate juice
- ✓ 1 cup water

Directions

- ✓ Combine all ingredients in a blender and mix until smooth.

Apple Smoothie

This refreshing smoothie is perfectly balanced between tart and sweet, thanks to Granny Smith apple, banana, orange juice, and honey.
Servings: 1 | Prep: 5 m | Total Time: 5 m

Ingredients

- ✓ 1 Granny Smith apple (about 8 ounces), peeled and chopped
- ✓ 1 banana (about 4 ounces), cut into chunks
- ✓ 1/2 cup orange juice
- ✓ 1/2 teaspoon pure vanilla extract
- ✓ 1 teaspoon honey
- ✓ 1 tablespoon golden flaxseed (optional)
- ✓ 1 cup ice

Directions

- ✓ Combine apple, banana, orange juice, vanilla, honey, flaxseed and ice in a blender. Puree on high until smooth. Serve.

Avocado Banana Smoothie

Try sipping your avocado -- this tropical-tasting avocado smoothie makes a satisfying breakfast or snack.

Servings: *4*

Ingredients

- ✓ 1 avocado
- ✓ 1 banana
- ✓ 1/2 cup nonfat plain Greek yogurt
- ✓ 1 1/2 cups fresh orange juice (from 3 oranges)
- ✓ 1/4 cup honey
- ✓ 2 1/2 to 3 cups ice

Directions

- ✓ In a blender, combine avocado, banana, yogurt, orange juice, honey, and ice. Blend until smooth. Serve immediately.

Avocado-Spinach Smoothie

This green smoothie gets its color from spinach, avocado, and a Granny Smith apple. It's packed with vitamins and contains six grams of filling fiber in each serving.

Servings: *2*

Ingredients

- ✓ 1 cup packed fresh spinach leaves

- ✓ 1 1/4 cups white grape juice or pear juice
- ✓ 1/2 avocado
- ✓ 1 Granny Smith apple, peeled and cut into 1-inch pieces
- ✓ 1 cup ice

Directions

- ✓ Blend spinach leaves, juice, avocado, apple, and ice.

Banana Blueberry Smoothie

You can substitute the blueberries with any other frozen fruit you like.
***Servings:** 2 | **Prep Time:** 5 mins| **Total Time:** 5 mins*

Ingredients

- ✓ 1 ripe banana
- ✓ 1 cup frozen blueberries
- ✓ 1 cup nonfat plain yogurt

Directions

1. In a blender, combine banana, blueberries, and yogurt.
2. Blend on high speed until smooth. Pour into two glasses; serve immediately.

Banana Nutmeg Smoothie

No need to skip breakfast. Try this banana-nutmeg smoothie to start your day, whether at home or on the go.
***Servings:** 2 | **Prep Time:** 5 mins | **Total Time:** 5 mins*

Ingredients

- ✓ 3 bananas, ripe but firm, broken into pieces
- ✓ 1/2 cup whole milk
- ✓ 1 cup low-fat vanilla yogurt
- ✓ 1 cup ice cubes

✓ 1/4 teaspoon nutmeg

Directions

1. In a blender, combine bananas, broken into pieces, with milk, and puree until smooth.
2. Add to the fruit mixture yogurt, ice cubes, and nutmeg, and blend until the ice is finely crushed and the drink is frothy. Serve immediately.

Banana-Oat Smoothie

Lean protein from milk and yogurt gives energy; soluble fiber from oats and banana boosts heart health.

Servings: 1

Ingredients

✓ 1/4 cup old-fashioned rolled oats
✓ 1/2 cup plain low-fat yogurt
✓ 1 banana, cut into thirds
✓ 1/2 cup fat-free milk
✓ 2 teaspoons honey
✓ 1/4 teaspoon ground cinnamon

Directions

✓ In a blender, combine oats, yogurt, banana, fat-free milk, honey, and cinnamon; puree until smooth. Serve immediately.

Banana-Yogurt Smoothie

A sneaky spoonful or two of flaxseeds is enough to help this morning smoothie make you feel like a star.

*Servings: 1 | **Prep:** 5 m | **Ready In:** 5 m*

Ingredients

- ✓ 2 teaspoons flaxseeds
- ✓ 1 medium banana (6 ounces)
- ✓ 1/2 cup low-fat plain yogurt
- ✓ 1 to 2 teaspoons honey
- ✓ 2/3 cup ice cubes

Directions

1. Place the flaxseeds in a blender and puree for 30 seconds until they are coarsely ground.
2. Add the banana, yogurt, honey, and ice cubes and puree until smooth and thick. Serve immediately.

Berry Orange Smoothie

Using sorbet instead of ice cream makes this creamy smoothie a satisfying dessert option as well as a delicious breakfast.

Servings: 2

Ingredients

- ✓ 1 orange, peel and pith removed with a sharp knife, quartered
- ✓ 1/2 cup low-fat plain yogurt
- ✓ 1/2 cup raspberry sorbet
- ✓ 1/2 cup 100 percent cranberry juice

Directions

- ✓ Blend orange, yogurt, sorbet, and juice.

Blackberry Yogurt Smoothies

This breakfast shake derives its deep flavor and color from blackberries, rich in vitamin C, mixed with a few spoonfuls of honey. Ground cardamom provides a counterbalance to the sweetness.

Servings: 4

Ingredients

- ✓ 12 ounces blackberries (3 cups)
- ✓ 1 cup plain low-fat yogurt
- ✓ 1 cup low-fat buttermilk
- ✓ 3 tablespoons honey
- ✓ 1 pinch ground cardamom

Directions

- ✓ Blend ingredients in a blender on high speed until smooth, and serve.

Blueberry Mint Smoothie

Avocado thickens this smoothie while lemon and orange juice provide citrus tang.

Serving: 1

Ingredients

- ✓ 1 cup frozen blueberries
- ✓ 1/2 avocado
- ✓ 1/4 cup orange juice
- ✓ 1/2 cup fresh mint leaves
- ✓ 1 teaspoon lemon juice
- ✓ 1/2 cup water

Directions

- ✓ Blend ingredients until smooth.

Blueberry Smoothie

Creamy from the yogurt and milk, and sweet from the blueberries and honey, this milk shake remains virtuous: The yogurt is low fat and the

milk is skim.
Serving: 2

Ingredients

- ✓ 1/2 cup blueberries
- ✓ 1/2 cup low-fat vanilla yogurt
- ✓ 1/2 cup skim milk
- ✓ 2 tablespoons honey
- ✓ 5 small ice cubes

Directions

- ✓ Mix all ingredients in a blender until smooth. Serve immediately in tall glasses.

Breakfast Smoothies

Any other ripe fruit, such as peaches or raspberries, can be substituted for the strawberries
Yield: *Makes 4 Eight-Ounce Smoothies*

Ingredients

- ✓ 1 1/2 cups (12 ounces) plain fat-free yogurt
- ✓ 3 to 4 bananas, peeled, cut into chunks
- ✓ 14 ounces strawberries, stems removed, roughly chopped to equal 3 cups
- ✓ 1/4 cup skim milk or soy milk
- ✓ 2 tablespoons honey
- ✓ 1 cup ice

Directions

- ✓ Gradually add all ingredients to the jar of a blender; puree until smooth. Serve.

Buttermilk Banana Smoothies

Sweetened with dried dates and a touch of honey, a banana smoothie
makes a quick, nutritious breakfast.
Servings: 2

Ingredients

- ✓ 1 cup low-fat buttermilk
- ✓ 2 ripe bananas, cut into 2-inch-thick rounds
- ✓ 11 dried pitted dates
- ✓ 1 teaspoon honey
- ✓ Pinch of salt
- ✓ 1 cup ice

Directions

- ✓ Blend all ingredients in a blender on high speed until mixture is smooth and ice is finely ground. Pour into two glasses.

Carrot Ginger Smoothie

Create your own juice bar at home with this energizing breakfast drink.
Servings: 2

Ingredients

- ✓ 1 banana, cut into chunks
- ✓ 1 cup ice cubes
- ✓ 1/2 cup bottled carrot juice
- ✓ 1/2 cup plain low-fat yogurt
- ✓ 3/4-inch piece peeled fresh ginger, coarsely chopped

Directions

- ✓ Puree all ingredients in a blender.

Carrot-Mango Smoothie

Shh...don't tell, but hidden inside this delicious smoothie is a ton of healthy vitamins including beta-carotene.

Servings: 2

Ingredients

- ✓ 1 mango, chopped (or 1 1/2 cups frozen mango chunks)
- ✓ 1 cup fresh carrot juice
- ✓ Dash freshly grated nutmeg
- ✓ 1/2 cup ice cubes (omit if using frozen mango)

Directions

- ✓ Puree ingredients in a blender until smooth.

Cherry Berry Tea Smoothies

Protein-rich tofu gives this drink a thick and creamy texture, and frozen blueberries, cherries, and grapes deliver deep flavor and additional antioxidants. Rooibos tea, grown in South Africa, adds an herbaceous sweetness to this fruit smoothie without the caffeine found in other teas.

Servings: 4

Ingredients

- ✓ 3/4 cup water
- ✓ 2 Rooibos tea bags
- ✓ 6 ounces silken tofu
- ✓ 10 ounces (2 cups) frozen sweet cherries
- ✓ 6 ounces (1 cup) frozen grapes
- ✓ 3 ounces (1/2 cup) frozen blueberries

Directions

1. Bring water to a simmer. Immediately remove from heat, and add tea bags. Let steep, uncovered, for 8 minutes.

Discard tea bags. Refrigerate tea until cold, about 40 minutes.

2. Puree tea, tofu, and fruit in a blender until smooth, and serve cold.

Citrus & Green Tea Detox Smoothie

Ingredients
- ✓ 1 navel orange
- ✓ 1 grapefruit
- ✓ The juice of half a lemon
- ✓ 1/2 cup of unsweetened green tea, chilled
- ✓ 1/2 cup of nonfat Greek yogurt
- ✓ 1/2 a frozen banana
- ✓ 1 cup of ice
- ✓ 1/2 tablespoon honey

Directions
1. Brew a cup of green tea, let it cool a bit then put it in the fridge to get nice and cold.
2. Peel and segment the orange and grapefruit, and add to the blender with the lemon juice, green tea, Greek yogurt, honey, and frozen banana.
3. Blend until just combined.
4. Add the ice and blend until fully crushed.
5. Taste-test to see if it is sweet enough for you. If not, add some more honey or agave

Citrus Smoothies

Ingredients
- ✓ 2 navel oranges

- ✓ 2 tangerines
- ✓ 4 bananas (frozen and slightly thawed or fresh)
- ✓ 1 meyer lemon
- ✓ 1 meyer lime
- ✓ 1 sour lemon (e.g. Eureka lemon)
- ✓ 1/4 cup milk
- ✓ 28 large ice cubes

Directions

1. Rinse and peel all fruits and add to blender. Add milk and top with ice cubes. Cover and blend until smooth. Smoothie should be thick.
2. Pour into glasses and enjoy!

Notes

- ✓ Smoothies are so versatile. Don't let one fruit you might not have on hand stop you from trying out this smoothie; just replace it with another.

Coconut Cherry Smoothie

Ingredients

- ✓ 2 cups frozen pitted cherries
- ✓ 1 cup coconut water
- ✓ 1 tablespoon lime juice

Directions

- ✓ Combine in a blender.

Cranberry Bliss Detox Smoothie

Cranberry Bliss Detox Smoothie. A tasty and cleansing drink to kick off the new year, or to enjoy any day!

Ingredients

- ✓ 2 apples, sliced, peel left on
- ✓ 2 pears, sliced, peel left on
- ✓ 1 lemon, peeled, cut in quarters, seeds removed
- ✓ 1 cup fresh cranberries
- ✓ 2 cups of filtered water (keep extra handy if needed)
- ✓ Sweetener of choice (my picks would be stevia, agave, or honey, in that order of preference)
- ✓ 4-6 Ice cubes (if you want a cooler smoothie)
- ✓ 1 Tablespoon turmeric
- ✓ 2 Teaspoons pumkin pie spice blend (optional) OR 2 teaspoons of cinnamon or 1 teaspoon of nutmeg

Directions

1. Blend ice, if using, and 1 cup of the filtered water together. Then add the spice powders and blend again. Add in all fruits and blend until smooth, adding water as necessary. Check the taste and adjust seasoning to taste. If it seems too thick, add more filtered water and re-blend.

2. Pour into festive glasses of your choice, and enjoy. I like to drink mine with a straw. You can store the smoothie, covered, in the fridge for two days, or freeze any leftover smoothie and enjoy another day.

Cranberry Detox Smoothie

A simple and delicious smoothie recipe that helps cleanse the body with anti-inflammatory vitamins, and minerals.

Ingredients

- ✓ 1 cup fresh frozen cranberries
- ✓ 1 apple, peeled and cored

- ✓ 1/2 cup almond milk (or milk of your choice)
- ✓ 1/2 cup water
- ✓ 1/2 teaspoon ground cinnamon
- ✓ 1/2 teaspoon ground turmeric

Directions

1. Add all the ingredients into a large blender and blend until smooth
2. Garnish with ground cinnamon and cranberries, if desired

Cucumber Blueberry Smoothie

This smoothie of cucumber and blueberries is brimming with antioxidants. It makes a great start to any day for breakfast or a mid afternoon snack.

Servings: 2

Ingredients

- ✓ 1 medium cucumber, peeled, seeded, and cut into 1-inch pieces
- ✓ 1 cup frozen blueberries
- ✓ 1 cup white grape juice or pear juice
- ✓ 1/2 cup low-fat plain yogurt

Directions

- ✓ Blend cucumber, blueberries, juice, and yogurt.

Detox Beet and Carrot Smoothie

Ingredients

- ✓ 1 carrot, peeled, sliced
- ✓ 1 beet, peeled, sliced
- ✓ ½ cup red grapes

- ✓ 1 clementine, peeled
- ✓ 1 slice of ginger, peeled, about the size of a quarter
- ✓ ½ cup green tea

Directions

1. Steam carrot and beet until just tender, about 10-15 minutes, depending on how thick your slices are. Let cool.
2. Place all ingredients in blender and blend until smooth.

Detox Blueberry Fruit Smoothie

Ingredients

- ✓ ½ cup frozen blueberries
- ✓ ¼ cup unsweetened cranberry juice
- ✓ 1-2 bananas

Directions

- ✓ Place all ingredients in a blender and blend until smooth.

Detox Cactus Smoothie

Ingredients

- ✓ 5 oz (1½ medium) cactus leaves, needles removed and chopped
- ✓ ½ (12 oz approx) fresh pineapple, cut in cubes and chilled
- ✓ 1½ banana, sliced and frozen
- ✓ oz (1 cup) plain Greek yogurt
- ✓ 2 limes, juiced
- ✓ 1½ cups almond milk
- ✓ ⅓ cup aloe vera water (optional)

Directions

1. Place all ingredients in the blender in the order shown.

2. Blend on low for 1 - 2 minutes, or until the cactus, pineapple, and banana are beginning to become well-blended. Slowly raise the speed to medium for one minute, then slowly raise to high, or until you see a vortex in the middle of the smoothie. Once you see the vortex, blend for another minute, or until creamy.

Detox Smoothie

This super detox smoothie is great for alkalizing your system. It is refreshing and packed with vitamins, minerals, fiber, and enzymes.

Ingredients
- ✓ 1 1/4 cups (310 ml) pineapple juice
- ✓ juice from 1/4 lemon
- ✓ handful fresh spinach leaves
- ✓ 1/4 teaspoons fresh grated ginger

Directions
1. Pour the juice into the blender
2. Add the lemon juice (Minus the seeds)
3. Grab a handful of fresh spinach leaves (They have rather mild flavor so they won't affect the final taste of your drink substantially)
4. And throw them into the blender
5. Peel the fresh ginger and grate it finely (We need just about 1/4 teaspoon)
6. And into the blender it goes as well
7. Blend till liquefied and green

Detoxifying Ginger Berry Beet Smoothie

Ingredients

- ✓ 1 small raw organic beet, peeled and chopped
- ✓ 1 cup coconut water (or filtered water)
- ✓ 1/2 cup ice
- ✓ 1/2 avocado, pitted
- ✓ 1 cup frozen raspberries
- ✓ 1 lime, juiced
- ✓ 1/4 cara cara or blood orange, peel removed
- ✓ 1/4 teaspoons fresh ginger root or ginger powder
- ✓ 1 tablespoon chia seeds
- ✓ 1-2 teaspoons fresh turmeric root or ground turmeric powder
- ✓ dash of sea salt
- ✓ dash of black pepper
- ✓ 1 packet stevia (optional)

Directions

Combine all ingredients in a high-speed blend until smooth.

Pour into two glasses and enjoy immediately!

Notes

- ✓ This smoothie can be made up to 1-2 days in advance or frozen for up to two months. Simply blend all ingredients and pour into a freezer safe container. Voila! A cleansing meal or snack ready on demand!

Easy Carrot-Mango Smoothie

We poached ripe plums with a vanilla bean, then pureed them with buttermilk and ice for a rich, tangy treat for breakfast or anytime.
Yield: *Makes One 8-Ounce Smoothie* | ***Prep***: *10 mins* | ***Total Time***: *10 mins*

Ingredients

- ✓ 1/2 cup carrot juice
- ✓ 1/4 cup frozen mango chunks
- ✓ 1/4 cup ice cubes

Directions

- ✓ Combine ingredients in a blender. Blend on medium speed until smooth, about 30 seconds. Pour into a tall glass (or travel mug) and enjoy immediately.

Fat Burning Green Smoothie

Servings: 6 | Total Time: 20 m

Ingredients

- ✓ 1 kiwi;
- ✓ 7-10 sprigs of parsley;
- ✓ 2 ring lemon (with zest);
- ✓ 5 mint leaves;
- ✓ 100 ml. of pure, non-carbonated water;
- ✓ 1-2 teaspoons of honey.

Directions

1. Grind in a blender kiwi. A little scratch can be left for decoration.
2. In the same blender put the parsley and rings of lemon zest.
3. In a blender add mint and sparkling water, and honey. Mix all into a homogeneous mass.
4. The finished cocktail will fill a glass, decorate with mint and a slice of kiwi. Enjoy.

Frozen Banana Smoothies

For babies age 1 and older, you may add 1 tablespoon honey and substitute 10 strawberries, stemmed and quartered, for the papaya.
Servings: *2* | **Yield:** *Makes 2 1/2 Cups*

Ingredients
- ✓ 2 bananas, peeled, sliced 1/2-inch-thick
- ✓ 1 cup papaya, peeled, seeded, and diced
- ✓ 2/3 cup orange juice

Directions
1. Place bananas and papaya in a single layer in resealable plastic bag; transfer to freezer for at least 1 hour.
2. Transfer frozen fruit to jar of blender; add orange juice, and puree until smooth.

Fruit Smoothie with Tofu

You can use a variety of fruits in this shake, so get creative.
Yield: *Makes 1 Two-Cups Serving*

Ingredients
- ✓ 6 ounces fruit, such as raspberries, blueberries, or mango
- ✓ 4 ounces silken tofu
- ✓ 2 tablespoons honey, or more to taste
- ✓ 1 cup ice

Directions
- ✓ Place all ingredients in a blender. Blend on high speed until the texture is creamy and ice has been finely ground. Serve immediately.

Fruit Smoothie

Even more cold-fighting nutrients can be added easily to this fruit smoothie by pureeing a banana, a kiwi, or 1/2 cup of yogurt with the other ingredients.

Yield*: Makes Two 1-Cup Servings*

Ingredients

- ✓ 2 navel oranges, peel and pith removed, cut into chunks
- ✓ 1 cup frozen raspberries
- ✓ 1 cup frozen blueberries

Directions

- ✓ Puree ingredients in a blender until smooth. Serve immediately.

Fruit and Yogurt Smoothie

An icy pear-and-yogurt smoothie is welcome and refreshing any time of the day.

Servings*: 2*

Ingredients

- ✓ 1 1/2 cups plain nonfat or low-fat yogurt
- ✓ 1/2 medium chopped peeled pear
- ✓ 1 small sliced banana
- ✓ 2 tablespoons protein powder
- ✓ 3/4 cup crushed ice (crush ice in a plastic bag with a rolling pin)

Directions

- ✓ Puree ingredients in a blender. Divide between 2 glasses and serve.

Ginger-Mint Detox Smoothie

Fresh, refreshing, and cleansing, this recipe makes an ideal "hangover" smoothie. If you've eaten or drank too much the night before, try sipping this smoothie in the morning to reboot and refresh your system.

Ingredients

- ✓ 1 cucumber, peeled
- ✓ 6-8 leaves romaine
- ✓ 1 cup coconut water, chilled
- ✓ 1 lime, freshly squeezed
- ✓ 1" piece fresh ginger
- ✓ 1 bunch fresh mint leaves

Directions

- ✓ Combine all ingredients in a blender until puree'd. Serve and enjoy immediately.

Golden Nectar Smoothie

This energizing drink can be served at breakfast, or over ice as a pick-me-up at any other time of day.
Servings: 4

Ingredients

- ✓ 2 cups freshly squeezed orange juice (about 6 oranges)
- ✓ 1/4 cup plus 1 tablespoon raw honey
- ✓ 1 tablespoon freshly squeezed lemon juice
- ✓ 2 teaspoons finely grated fresh ginger
- ✓ 2 ripe bananas

Directions

- ✓ In a blender, puree all ingredients until smooth. Serve immediately.

Green Ginger-Peach Smoothie

Ingredients

- ✓ 2 handfuls baby spinach
- ✓ 1 teaspoon grated peeled fresh ginger
- ✓ 2 cups frozen sliced peaches
- ✓ 2 teaspoons honey
- ✓ 1 1/4 cups water

Directions

- ✓ Toss into blender.

Green Machine Smoothie

Detox Cred: Starting the day with this nutrient-dense elixir is a delicious way to charge your system with nutrients. Dark leafy greens are extremely alkalizing, meaning they foster a more neutral body environment for better functioning enzymes, compared with acid-forming foods like meats and dairy.

Serving: 2

Ingredients

- ✓ 6 romaine leaves, chopped
- ✓ 4 kale leaves, chopped
- ✓ 1/2 cup fresh parsley sprigs
- ✓ 1/2 cup chopped pineapple
- ✓ 1/2 cup chopped mango
- ✓ 1 inch fresh ginger, peeled and chopped

Directions

- ✓ Combine romaine, kale, parsley, pineapple, mango, ginger, and 1 1/2 cups water in a blender and blend until smooth.

Green Smoothie With Sea Buckthorn

Ingredients

- ✓ 40 ml sea buckthorn mousse (approx. 5 tbsp)
- ✓ 1 banana
- ✓ 1 orange or 2 tangerines
- ✓ 1 slice of fresh pineapple
- ✓ 1 large handful of fresh spinach
- ✓ 1 celery stick (optional)
- ✓ 1 cm fresh ginger
- ✓ 1/4 tsp ground turmeric
- ✓ a small pinch of ground black pepper *
- ✓ 1 C filtered water

Directions

1. Peel and cut the pineapple. Wash the spinach and celery stick. Peel and grate the ginger. Prepare all the other ingredients. If your blender can handle mixing the whole orange / tangerin just divide them into pieces, if not, then squeeze the juice and use only the juice for the smoothie.
2. Blend all ingredients until smooth and consume immediately.

Hearty Fruit and Oat Smoothie

Servings: 4

Ingredients

- ✓ 1 cup quartered strawberries
- ✓ 1 sliced banana
- ✓ 1/4 cup raw almonds
- ✓ 1/2 cup old-fashioned oats
- ✓ 1 cup low-fat vanilla yogurt
- ✓ 1 teaspoon maple syrup

Directions

- ✓ Toss into blender.

Heavy Metal Detox Oatmeal Smoothie

Ingredients

- ✓ ¼ C. leftover oatmeal, quinoameal, or buchwheatmeal
- ✓ 1 C. Almond coconut milk or skim milk
- ✓ ½ C. Cocunut water
- ✓ ½ C. Green Apple (1/2 C.)
- ✓ ¼ C. Fresh parsley
- ✓ ¼ C. Fresh cilantro
- ✓ 1 Tbsp. Raw honey
- ✓ 3-4 Ice cubes

Directions

- ✓ Combine all ingredients in a blender. Blend on high until well blended and smooth. Transfer to a glass and enjoy.

Notes

- ✓ This drink is best when consumed early in the morning on an empty stomach.

Holiday Detox Apple Strawberry Smoothie

Ingredients

- ✓ 1 apple (I used breaburn and left the skin on)
- ✓ 5 large frozen strawberries (if yours are small use 6-7)
- ✓ ½ a frozen banana
- ✓ 2 handfuls of ice
- ✓ ¾-1 cup coconut water (I use ZICO brand)

Directions

1. Add everything into the blender and blend until smooth
2. This makes about 16 oz.
3. Serves 2 small drinks or 1 large drink! ;-)
4. (If seeds bother you, you can strain this but I DO NOT the strawberry seeds are SO small and if your blender is good you won't even notice them!)

Immune-Boosting Strawberry Smoothie

Ingredients

- ✓ 1/2 frozen banana
- ✓ 1 cup frozen strawberries
- ✓ 1/2 medium beet, cold or frozen (see notes)
- ✓ Heaping 1/2 tsp. fresh grated ginger
- ✓ 1 cup water or coconut water
- ✓ 1/2 tsp. lime juice
- ✓ 3-4 ice cubes (or more if needed)

Directions

- ✓ Combine all ingredients in a blender and blend until smooth. Add ice until desired consistency is reached!

Kiwi Super Green Smoothie

Ingredients

- ✓ 2 kiwis (peeled)
- ✓ 1 lime (juiced)
- ✓ 1 lemon (juiced)
- ✓ 1 cup coconut water
- ✓ 4 oz orange juice
- ✓ Ice
- ✓ 1 sprig of parsley
- ✓ Small handful of baby spinach (for better digestion, slightly steam beforehand)
- ✓ 1 tablespoon chia seed
- ✓ 1/2 teaspoons ground ginger
- ✓ Pinch of sea salt
- ✓ Optional 1 teaspoons maple syrup or honey

Directions

- ✓ Blend and serve! I used about 1 cup ice.

Notes

1. Feel free to let the chia seed thicken by letting it sit in fridge for 30 minutes after you blend.
2. You can also use 1-2 tablespoon of vegan protein if you'd like to thicken it.

Low Carb Green Smoothie

These greens will cleanse and refresh your body.

Ingredients

- ✓ 1 cup coconut water
- ✓ 1Tablespoon almond butter
- ✓ ¼ cup wheat grass
- ✓ 2 cups spinach

- ✓ 1 scoop high quality, low carb chocolate protein
- ✓ 1 inch slice of banana
- ✓ Optional pinch of Stevia
- ✓ ½ cup ice

Directions

- ✓ Combine all the ingredients in your high speed blender then blend on high for a full minute, or until the tiny pieces of spinach have disappeared and the smoothie turns a brilliant shade of green.

Nutrition

- ✓ Calories: 155
- ✓ Fat: 4 g
- ✓ Carbohydrates: 15 g
- ✓ Sodium: 105 mg
- ✓ Fiber: 2 g
- ✓ Protein: 15 g

Mango and Yogurt Smoothie

Ingredients

- ✓ 1/4 teaspoon ground cinnamon
- ✓ 1 1/2 cups low-fat plain yogurt
- ✓ 2 1/2 cups frozen mango chunks
- ✓ 1 tablespoon honey
- ✓ Juice from half lime

Directions

- ✓ Toss into blender.

Mango Green Tea Detox Smoothie

This mango and green tea detox smoothie is full of nutrients and natural antioxidants - perfect for a detox or cleanse!

Ingredients

- ✓ Green Tea Concentrate
- ✓ 3 Green Tea Bags
- ✓ 1 Cup Hot Water
- ✓ The Rest of the Smoothie
- ✓ 1 Cup Frozen Mango
- ✓ ½ Cup Frozen Pineapple
- ✓ 1 Cup Fresh Kale

Directions

1. To make the green tea concentrate, steep green tea bags in hot water for 10 minutes.
2. In a blender, combine green tea concentrate, fruit, and kale, and blend until smooth.
3. Pour into glasses and serve!

Mango Lassi Smoothie

This smoothie showcases the flavors of a mango lassi, a traditional Indian yogurt-based drink. Our version calls for fresh mango, cinnamon, and a touch of salt to balance the sweetness.
Serving: 4 | Prep: 5 m | Ready In: 5 m

Ingredients

- ✓ 2 cups chopped mango (from 1 large peeled, pitted mango)
- ✓ 1/2 cup ice
- ✓ 1 cup plain whole-milk yogurt
- ✓ 2 tablespoons sugar, or to taste
- ✓ Pinch of ground cinnamon
- ✓ Pinch of coarse salt

Directions

- ✓ Combine mango, ice, yogurt, sugar, cinnamon, and salt in a blender; blend until smooth, 1 minute. Serve immediately.

Mango Tahini Smoothie

The tahini gives this smoothie a distinctive flavor.
Servings: 1

Ingredients

- ✓ 1 cup slightly thawed frozen mango
- ✓ 1 tablespoon tahini
- ✓ 1 tablespoon lime juice
- ✓ 1/2 cup water

Directions

- ✓ Blend ingredients until smooth.

Matcha Mango Pineapple Smoothie

Ingredients

- ✓ 1.25 teaspoons matcha green tea (I use DavidsTea's Matcha Matsu)
- ✓ 1 scoop protein powder
- ✓ some honey
- ✓ 1 c frozen mango chunks
- ✓ 1 tablespoon pineapple juice
- ✓ 1 c pineapple
- ✓ 1/2 to 1 c water (depending on how thick you like your smoothies)

Directions

✓ If you're using fresh fruit, chop it all up then toss it all in a blender! Done!

Melon, Mint, and Cucumber Smoothie

Refreshing and hydrating, this smoothie is a great way to get in a few extra helpings of fruits and veggies.
***Serving**: 2*

Ingredients

✓ 2 cups chopped honeydew
✓ 1 cup chopped English cucumber
✓ 12 fresh mint leaves
✓ 2-4 tablespoons fresh lime juice, to taste
✓ 1 teaspoon honey

Directions

✓ Puree ingredients in a blender until smooth.

Nectarine-Yogurt Smoothie

Using almond milk is less calories than skim milk and provides distinctive flavor to this smoothie.
***Servings**: 2*

Ingredients

✓ 2 medium nectarines (10 ounces total), pitted and quartered, or 8 ounces frozen peaches
✓ 1/2 cup unsweetened almond milk
✓ 1 tablespoon honey
✓ 1/3 cup nonfat plain Greek yogurt

✓ 1/2 cup ice (if using fresh nectarines)

Directions

✓ In a blender, combine nectarines or peaches, almond milk, honey, yogurt, and ice. Blend until smooth.

Oat Coconut Smoothie

*Serving: 1 | **Prep**: 5 m | **Ready In**: 5 m*

Ingredients

✓ 1/2 banana
✓ 1/4 cup old-fashioned rolled oats
✓ 1/3 cup Greek yogurt
✓ 2 tablespoons coconut oil
✓ 1 tablespoon honey
✓ 1/3 cup freshly squeezed orange juice
✓ 1/2 cup ice

Directions

✓ In a blender, combine banana, oats, yogurt, coconut oil, honey, orange juice, and ice. Puree until smooth. Transfer to a tall glass and drink immediately.

Papaya-Ginger Smoothie

Papaya has a slight muskiness that makes it a good partner for both mild and assertive ingredients. Coupling it with mint gives this quick-to-fix smoothie a bright, clean taste.
Servings: 4

Ingredients

✓ 2 1/2 cups papaya (Solo or Mexican) chunks

- ✓ 1 cup ice cubes
- ✓ 2/3 cup nonfat plain yogurt
- ✓ 1 tablespoon finely chopped peeled fresh ginger
- ✓ 1 tablespoon honey
- ✓ Juice of 2 lemons
- ✓ 16 fresh mint leaves, plus 4 sprigs for garnish

Directions

1. Refrigerate papaya until very cold, at least 1 hour or overnight.
2. Blend papaya, ice, yogurt, ginger, honey, and lemon juice in a blender. Add up to 1/4 cup water, 1 tablespoon at a time, until mixture is smooth and thinned to desired consistency. Blend in mint leaves. Garnish with mint sprigs.

Peach, Berry, and Spinach Smoothie

Using frozen peaches and blackberries instead of fresh in this smoothie lets you have a bit of summer in the middle of a snowstorm.

Servings: 2

Ingredients

- ✓ 1 cup fresh or frozen peach slices
- ✓ 1/2 cup fresh or frozen blackberries
- ✓ 1 cup packed fresh spinach leaves
- ✓ 1 1/2 cups white grape juice
- ✓ 1/2 cup ice (if using fresh fruit)

Directions

- ✓ Blend peach slices, blackberries, spinach leaves, grape juice, and ice (if using fresh fruit).

Peanut-Banana Espresso Smoothie

Your morning routine just became portable. Creamy peanut butter and banana come together with espresso powder in this smoothie that packs a punch.
Serving: 2

Ingredients

- ✓ 1 cup low-fat milk
- ✓ 1 tablespoon instant espresso powder
- ✓ 1/4 cup natural creamy peanut butter
- ✓ 1 ripe banana, cut into thirds
- ✓ 1 cup ice

Directions

- ✓ Blend milk, espresso powder, peanut butter, banana, and ice.

Pineapple and Ginger Smoothie

Drink up! The fresh ginger in this tropical pineapple smoothie has cancer-fighting powers.
Servings: 2

Ingredients

- ✓ 1 cup fresh or frozen pineapple, cut into 1-inch pieces
- ✓ 1 inch piece fresh ginger, peeled and minced
- ✓ 1/2 cup low-fat plain yogurt
- ✓ 1 cup pineapple juice
- ✓ 1/8 teaspoon ground cinnamon
- ✓ 1/2 cup ice (if using fresh pineapple)

Directions

- ✓ Blend pineapple, ginger, yogurt, pineapple juice, cinnamon, and ice (if using fresh pineapple).

Pineapple Banana Smoothie

This is a quick and tasty way to start your morning.
Servings: 2 | Prep Time: 5 mins| Total Time: 5 mins

Ingredients

- ✓ 1 8-ounce can crushed pineapple in juice
- ✓ 1 banana
- ✓ 1 6-ounce container plain nonfat yogurt
- ✓ 1/2 cup ice cubes
- ✓ Grated nutmeg

Directions

- ✓ In a blender, combine crushed pineapple with juice, banana, yogurt, and ice cubes. Puree until smooth. Sprinkle with grated nutmeg and serve.

Plum Persimmon Green Smoothie

Ingredients

- ✓ 1/2 a green apple, sliced
- ✓ 1 black plum, sliced
- ✓ 1/2 a persimmon, sliced
- ✓ 2 satsuma oranges, peeled and separated
- ✓ Small nugget of ginger, as desired
- ✓ Juice of 1/3 a large lemon
- ✓ 1 cup fresh spinach
- ✓ Handful of kale (1/4-1/2 cup)

- ✓ 4 ice cubes

Directions

- ✓ Peel and chop fruit and vegetables as directed and add to a blender. Blend until smooth. Add ice last and blend again.

Pom-Berry-Banana Smoothie

Get your morning off to a bright start with this vibrant smoothie bursting with tart pomegranate juice and mixed berries.

Servings: 2

Ingredients

- ✓ 1 orange, peel and pith removed with a sharp knife, quartered
- ✓ 1 cup frozen mixed berries
- ✓ 1 ripe banana, cut into thirds
- ✓ 1 cup 100 percent pomegranate juice

Directions

- ✓ Blend orange, berries, banana, and pomegranate juice.

Pomegranate Smoothie

Antioxidant-rich berries, fruit juice, and protein-packed tofu and pomegranate make a nourishing breakfast.

Serving: 2

Ingredients

- ✓ 1/3 cup silken tofu (about 3 ounces)
- ✓ 1 cup frozen mixed berries
- ✓ 1/2 cup pomegranate juice

- ✓ 1 to 2 teaspoons honey
- ✓ 1/4 cup ice cubes

Directions

- ✓ In a blender, combine tofu, berries, juice, honey, and ice cubes; puree until smooth. Serve immediately.

Power Protein Smoothie

Smoothies offer incredible versatility: You can use whatever's in season. The berries combined with pomegranate juice give this drinkable breakfast an extra antioxidant boost.
Servings: 2 | Prep Time: 5 minutes | Total Time: 5 minutes

Ingredients

- ✓ 2 cups mixed berries (fresh or frozen)
- ✓ 1 cup silken tofu
- ✓ 1/4 cup pomegranate juice
- ✓ 2 to 3 tablespoons honey
- ✓ 2 tablespoons ground flaxseed
- ✓ 1 teaspoon finely grated peeled ginger

Directions

- ✓ In a blender, combine berries, tofu, pomegranate juice, 2 tablespoons honey, flaxseed, and ginger. Blend until smooth, 15 to 20 seconds. Adjust the sweetness if neccessary.

Spinach Avocado Smoothie

This better-for-you blend with spinach and avocado is naturally delicious and nutritious and is a superb way to start your day.
Serving: 2| Prep: 5 m | Ready In: 5 m

Ingredients

- ✓ 1 cup packed spinach leaves
- ✓ 1 1/4 cups white grape juice or pear juice
- ✓ 1/2 avocado
- ✓ 1 Granny Smith apple, peeled and cut into 1-inch pieces
- ✓ 1 cup ice

Directions

- ✓ Blend spinach, juice, avocado, apple, and ice.

Stay-Young Smoothie

For a healthy breakfast, try this invigorating blend of berries, green tea, flaxseed, and low-fat yogurt. That's what we'd call smooth.
Yield: *Makes One 14-Ounce Smoothie*

Ingredients

- ✓ 1/2 cup frozen organic blueberries
- ✓ 1/2 cup frozen organic strawberries
- ✓ 1/2 cup chilled green tea, unsweetened
- ✓ 3/4 cup plain low-fat organic yogurt
- ✓ 2 tablespoons ground flaxseed
- ✓ Turbinado sugar or other natural sweetener to taste

Directions

- ✓ Combine all ingredients in an electric blender and blend on medium speed until smooth, about 20 seconds. Garnish with fresh berries and serve.

Strawberry Soy Smoothie

Read the soy milk label, and choose one that is low in sugar and fortified with calcium.

Servings: 2

Ingredients

- ✓ 1 ripe banana, thickly sliced
- ✓ 2 cup strawberries, hulled
- ✓ 1 cup soy milk
- ✓ 2 tablespoons honey

Directions

- ✓ In a blender, combine ripe banana, strawberries, soy milk, and honey. Puree until smooth.

Strawberry, Mango, and Yogurt Smoothie

You can use fresh or frozen fruit in this smoothie and substitute orange juice for the apple.

Servings: 2

Ingredients

- ✓ 1 1/4 cups apple juice
- ✓ 1 cup low-fat plain yogurt
- ✓ 1 cup fresh or frozen strawberries
- ✓ 2 cups fresh or frozen mango chunks

Directions

- ✓ In a blender, combine all ingredients and puree until smooth.

Strawberry-Coconut Smoothie

This smoothie gets a flavor boost from light coconut milk.

Servings: 1

Ingredients

- ✓ 1 cup slightly thawed frozen strawberries
- ✓ 1 banana
- ✓ 2 tablespoons light coconut milk
- ✓ 1 teaspoon lemon juice
- ✓ 3/4 cup water

Directions

- ✓ Blend all ingredients until smooth.

Strawberry-Grapefruit Smoothie

Start your morning with this zingy, antioxidant-packed smoothie.
Yield*: Makes Three 1 3/4-Cup Servings*

Ingredients

- ✓ 1 grapefruit, peeled, seeded, and chopped
- ✓ 2 cups hulled fresh or frozen strawberries
- ✓ 1 sweet apple (such as Honeycrisp or Pink Lady), cored and chopped
- ✓ 1 inch fresh ginger, peeled and chopped

Directions

- ✓ Combine all ingredients, plus 1 cup water, in a blender and process until smooth.

Superfood Detox Smoothie

Prep*: 5 m |* **Ready In***: 5 m*

Ingredients

- ✓ 1 Cup Fresh Pineapple
- ✓ 1 Cup Frozen Blueberries

- ✓ Juice from 1 Grapefruit
- ✓ 2 tablespoon Goji Berries, soaked in hot water for 5 minutes

Directions

1. Soak the goji berries in hot water for about five minutes, to soften. Once they're soft, drain the water and stick the berries in the blender.
2. Add in the pineapple, blueberries, and grapefruit juice, and blend on high until smooth and creamy.
3. Serve in glasses and enjoy!

Superfood Smoothie

Four healthful "superfoods" -- soy, blueberries, yogurt, and orange -- make this a nutrient-packed breakfast or snack.

Serving: 1

Ingredients

- ✓ 3/4 cup fresh or frozen blueberries
- ✓ 1/2 cup ice
- ✓ 1/2 cup plain low-fat regular or Greek yogurt
- ✓ 2 tablespoons fresh orange juice
- ✓ 2 tablespoons soymilk
- ✓ 1 tablespoon honey

Directions

- ✓ In a blender, combine all ingredients. Blend until smooth, scraping down sides of blender as needed. Serve immediately.

Tropical Blueberry Smoothie

Ingredients

- ✓ 2 teaspoons sugar
- ✓ 1 cup chopped pineapple
- ✓ 1 1/2 cups frozen blueberries
- ✓ 1 orange, seeded and cut into quarters
- ✓ 1/2–3/4 cup water

Directions

- ✓ Toss into blender.

Vanilla, Plum, and Buttermilk Smoothie

We poached ripe plums with a vanilla bean, then pureed them with buttermilk and ice for a rich, tangy treat for breakfast or anytime.

Servings: 6

Ingredients

- ✓ 2 cups sugar
- ✓ 1 vanilla bean, halved with scraped seeds
- ✓ 5 plums, quartered, pitted
- ✓ 1/2 cup buttermilk
- ✓ 1 1/2 cups small ice cubes

Directions

1. Put 4 cups water, sugar, and halved vanilla bean with scraped seeds into a large saucepan. Bring to a boil over medium-high heat, stirring until sugar has dissolved. Add plums. Reduce heat to medium-low, and simmer until plums are tender, about 15 minutes. Using a slotted spoon, transfer plums to a plate to cool completely; remove bean, and discard poaching liquid.

2. Puree cooled plums in a blender. Add buttermilk and small ice cubes; blend until smooth.

Winter Smoothie

This healthy citrus smoothie is a satisfying alternative to a heavy breakfast. It's simple to make: Alternate layers or orange and pineapple slush, and mix yogurt and sliced bananas.
Servings: 4

Ingredients
- ✓ 2 1/2 cups pineapple juice
- ✓ 2 1/2 cups freshly squeezed orange juice, plus orange sections for garnish (optional)
- ✓ 3/4 cup plain yogurt
- ✓ 1 banana, peeled and halved
- ✓ 3 tablespoons honey
- ✓ 1/4 teaspoon ground cinnamon, plus more for garnish

Directions
1. Fill one ice-cube tray with pineapple juice and another tray with orange juice. Place in the freezer until frozen, several hours or overnight. Place yogurt, banana, honey, and cinnamon in the jar of a blender, and process until smooth. Transfer to a bowl, and set aside. Rinse blender, and fill with pineapple ice cubes and remaining pineapple juice. Process until smooth.
2. Divide among four glasses, top with reserved yogurt mixture, and place in the freezer. Meanwhile, process the orange-juice cubes with the remaining orange juice. Remove filled glasses from freezer, and top with orange-juice slush. Garnish each glass with additional cinnamon and an orange section, if desired. Serve immediately.

Yogurt Pistachio Smoothies

Servings: 6

Ingredients

- ✓ 2 cups plain yogurt
- ✓ 1/2 cup water
- ✓ 1 1/2 teaspoons finely grated fresh ginger
- ✓ 1/2 cup salted pistachios
- ✓ 1/4 teaspoon freshly ground pepper
- ✓ 4 ice cubes
- ✓ 1/4 cup finely chopped pistachios

Directions

- ✓ Blend yogurt, water, ginger, salted pistachios, pepper, and ice cubes until smooth. Divide among glasses. Garnish with finely chopped pistachios.

Four: Mocktail Recipes

* * *

There's no mocking these alcohol-free faves. They're fun,
sometimes fizzy, always 5-star refreshing.

Abstinence on the Beach

"To die for! When I entertain a crowd, I make a non-alcoholic base, then have decanter of equal parts vodka and peach schnapps next to the pitcher so people can liven it up if desired."
***Servings**: 12 | **Prep**: 10 mins | **Total time**:2 h 10 mins*

Ingredients

- ✓ 1 (12 fluid ounce) can frozen concentrated grapefruit juice
- ✓ 1 (12 fluid ounce) can frozen cranberry juice concentrate
- ✓ 1/4 cup coconut milk
- ✓ 9 cups cold water

Directions

1. In a 6 quart container combine concentrated grapefruit juice, concentrated cranberry juice and water. Put about 1 cup of juice and coconut milk in food processor or blender. Blend until smooth and pour back into main juice mixture. Stir to incorporate.
2. Chill at least 2 hours. Serve in punch bowl or pitcher.

Nutritional Information

- ✓ Calories: 123 kcal 6%
- ✓ Fat: 1.1 g 2%
- ✓ Carbs: 28.5g 9%
- ✓ Protein: 0.7 g 1%
- ✓ Cholesterol: 0 mg 0%
- ✓ Sodium: 3 mg < 1%

Alcohol-Free Mint Julep

*"An alcohol FREE mint julep for you non-drinkers out there.... now you
don't have to drink water and can enjoy the classic mint julep with a
slight twist while watching the Kentucky Derby!"*
Servings: 2 | **Prep**: 15 m | **Cook**: 10 m | **Ready In**: 1 h 25 m

Ingredients

- ✓ 1/4 cup water
- ✓ 1/4 cup white sugar
- ✓ 1 tablespoon chopped fresh mint leaves
- ✓ 2 cups crushed ice
- ✓ 1/2 cup prepared lemonade
- ✓ Fresh mint sprigs, for garnish

Directions

1. In a small saucepan, combine the water, sugar and 1 tablespoon of chopped mint. Stir and bring to a boil. Cook until sugar has dissolved, then remove from heat and set aside to cool. After about an hour, strain out mint leaves.

2. Fill 2 cups or frozen goblets with crushed ice. Pour 1/2 of the lemonade into each glass and top with a splash of the sugar syrup. Garnish each with a mint sprig and a straw. Serve on a silver platter.

Nutritional Information

- ✓ Calories: 122 kcal 6%
- ✓ Fat: 0 g < 1%
- ✓ Carbs: 31.6g 10%
- ✓ Protein: 0.1 g < 1%
- ✓ Cholesterol: 0 mg 0%
- ✓ Sodium: 7 mg < 1%

Alcohol-Free Mojitos

*"These are great for the kids or for anyone who wants a refreshing
alcohol-free drink."*
Servings: 14 | **Prep**: 15 m | **Ready In**: 15 m

Ingredients
- ✓ 2 cups water
- ✓ 1 1/2 cups white sugar
- ✓ 2 cups mint leaves, chopped
- ✓ 2 cups lime sherbet, softened
- ✓ 1 cup lime juice 1 cup water
- ✓ 8 cups club soda
- ✓ Lime slices for garnish

Directions
1. Combine 2 cups water and the sugar in a microwave-safe bowl; heat in microwave on High for 5 minutes. Stir the mint into the water; let stand for 5 minutes. Strain and discard the mint leaves from the syrup; set aside.
2. Stir the lime sherbet, lime juice, and 1 cup water together in a large pitcher until well combined. Pour the mint-infused syrup into the mixture. Add club soda and stir. Serve over ice. Garnish with lime slices.

Nutritional Information
- ✓ Calories: 120 kcal 6%
- ✓ Fat: 0.5 g < 1%
- ✓ Carbs: 30.3g 10%
- ✓ Protein: 0.5 g < 1%
- ✓ Cholesterol: 1 mg < 1%
- ✓ Sodium: 16 mg < 1%

Apple Julep

"A great blend of juices that is great with breakfast or anytime."
***Servings**: 6 | **Prep**: 5 m | **Ready In**: 5 m*

Ingredients

- ✓ 1 quart apple juice
- ✓ 1 cup orange juice
- ✓ 1 cup pineapple juice
- ✓ 1/4 cup lemon juice
- ✓ 1 sprig fresh mint leaves

Directions

- ✓ In a large pitcher, stir together the apple juice, orange juice, pineapple juice and lemon juice. Mix and pour into glasses full of ice to serve. Garnish each serving with a mint leaf.

Nutritional Information

- ✓ Calories: 121 kcal 6%
- ✓ Fat: 0.3 g < 1%
- ✓ Carbs: 29.8g 10%
- ✓ Protein: 0.6 g 1%
- ✓ Cholesterol: 0 mg 0%
- ✓ Sodium: 6 mg < 1%

Banana Bonkers

"Wonderful tall, cool banana drink that is great on the deck in the hot afternoon. Kids love this also. Optionally, you can mix in 3 eggs which have been whipped in the blender."
***Servings**: 6 | **Prep**: 20 m | **Ready In**: 20 m*

Ingredients

- ✓ 3 bananas
- ✓ 3 cups fresh grapefruit juice
- ✓ 2 cups lemon sherbet
- ✓ 1 cup crushed ice

Directions

- ✓ Puree bananas in a blender or food processor. In a gallon pitcher combine pureed bananas, grapefruit juice, lemon sherbet and crushed ice. Stir and serve.

Nutritional Information

- ✓ Calories: 181 kcal 9%
- ✓ Fat: 0.3 g < 1%
- ✓ Carbs: 45.5g 15%
- ✓ Protein: 1.3 g 3%
- ✓ Cholesterol: 0 mg 0%
- ✓ Sodium: 6 mg < 1%

Berry Refresher

"This recipe is a perfect refresher for a hot summer day or to quench a raging thirst! Absolutely delicious! To make it thick, simply use berries frozen!"

*Servings: 4 | **Prep**: 10 m | **Ready In**: 10 m*

Ingredients

- ✓ 1 cup apple juice
- ✓ 1 cup orange juice
- ✓ 1/3 cup milk
- ✓ 1 tablespoon honey
- ✓ 2 frozen strawberries, thawed
- ✓ 1/3 cup frozen raspberries, thawed
- ✓ 2/3 cup frozen blueberries, thawed

- ✓ 3 cubes ice

Directions
- ✓ Place the apple juice, orange juice, milk, honey, strawberries, raspberries, blueberries, and ice cubes in a blender. Blend until slushy. Serve cold.

Nutritional Information
- ✓ Calories: 120 kcal 6%
- ✓ Fat: 0.8 g 1%
- ✓ Carbs: 28g 9%
- ✓ Protein: 1.4 g 3%
- ✓ Cholesterol: 2 mg < 1%
- ✓ Sodium: 12 mg < 1%

Cherry Lime Ricky

"Discover the refreshing pleasure of this old-time soda fountain favorite."
Servings: 1 | Prep: 5 m | Ready In: 5 m

Ingredients
- ✓ 1/2 cup tart cherry juice
- ✓ Juice of 1 lime
- ✓ 1 packet Sweet'N Low granulated sugar substitute
- ✓ Club soda
- ✓ Lime wedge, for garnish (optional)

Directions
1. In a measuring cup, combine the cherry juice, lime juice, and Sweet'N Low. Stir to dissolve the Sweet'N Low.
2. Fill a tall glass with ice. Pour in the cherry juice mixture. Top with the club soda. Serve with a straw, garnished with the lime wedge, if desired.

Nutritional Information
- ✓ Calories: 81 kcal 4%

- ✓ Fat: 0.5 g < 1%
- ✓ Carbs: 21.2g 7%
- ✓ Protein: 0.7 g 1%
- ✓ Cholesterol: 0 mg 0%
- ✓ Sodium: 23 mg < 1%

Chinese Firebolt

"My stepdad and I have a favorite drink that we created, and it's really amazing! It's delicious and fizzy, anyone would love it. Named after the fierce dragon in Harry Potter and the Goblet of Fire, (I know, we're HP freaks) it's great for a non-alcoholic drink at a party!"

Servings: 1 | Prep: 5 m | Ready In: 5 m

Ingredients
- ✓ 1 tablespoon cherry grenadine syrup
- ✓ 1 tablespoon lime juice
- ✓ 1 (12 fluid ounce) can or bottle cola soft drink (such as Coke®)
- ✓ 1 strip of lemon zest, for garnish

Directions
- ✓ Plour the grenadine and lime juice into a tall glass. Pour in the cola to mix. Float a strip of lemon zest on top to garnish.

Nutritional Information
- ✓ Calories: 211 kcal 11%
- ✓ Fat: 0 g < 1%
- ✓ Carbs: 53.6g 17%
- ✓ Protein: 0.1 g < 1%
- ✓ Cholesterol: 0 mg 0%
- ✓ Sodium: 21 mg < 1%

Cool Watermelon Slushes

"A Thailand watermelon slushie that is sweetened with honey. You may use sugar if you wish though."
***Servings**: 4 | **Prep**: 3 m | **Cook**: 3 m | **Ready In**: 6 m*

Ingredients

- ✓ 6 ice cubes
- ✓ 2 cups cubed seeded watermelon
- ✓ 1 teaspoon honey

Directions

- ✓ Place the ice cubes into a blender. Cover, and pulse until crushed. Add the watermelon and blend for about 1 minute, until slushy. Add the honey, and blend for about 10 seconds.

Nutritional Information

- ✓ Calories: 28 kcal 1%
- ✓ Fat: 0.1 g < 1%
- ✓ Carbs: 7.3g 2%
- ✓ Protein: 0.5 g < 1%
- ✓ Cholesterol: 0 mg 0%
- ✓ Sodium: 2 mg < 1%

Cran-Dandy Cooler

"A carbonated cranberry and pineapple refreshing cooler."
***Servings**: 8 | **Prep**: 10 m | **Ready In**: 10 m*

Ingredients

- ✓ 2 cups cranberry juice

- ✓ 1 cup pineapple juice
- ✓ 1 cup orange juice
- ✓ 1 (4 ounce) jar maraschino cherries
- ✓ 2 tablespoons lemon juice
- ✓ 1 (12 fluid ounce) can or bottle ginger ale
- ✓ 1 orange, sliced in rounds

Directions

- ✓ In a gallon pitcher combine cranberry juice, pineapple juice, orange juice, cherry juice and lemon juice. Just before serving, slowly add ginger ale; stir to blend. Serve over ice in cups or glasses. Garnish with cherry and orange slices.

Nutritional Information

- ✓ Calories: 107 kcal 5%
- ✓ Fat: 0.2 g < 1%
- ✓ Carbs: 26.5g 9%
- ✓ Protein: 0.6 g 1%
- ✓ Cholesterol: 0 mg 0%
- ✓ Sodium: 8 mg < 1%

Exotic Fruit Drink

"This contains three different fruit juices that everyone will love! Use your imagination and come up with different combinations!"
Servings: 4 | **Prep**: 5 m | **Cook**: 2 m | **Ready In**: 2 h 5 m

Ingredients

- ✓ 1 cup orange juice
- ✓ 1 cup cranberry juice
- ✓ 1/2 cup lemon juice
- ✓ 1 (32 fluid ounce) bottle carbonated water

Directions

1. Put the orange juice, cranberry juice and lemon juice in 3 separate cups. Without mixing the juices, pour them into ice cube trays and freeze.

2. When frozen, place one of each juice cube into a tall glass and fill the glass with carbonated water.

Nutritional Information

✓ Calories: 70 kcal 3%

✓ Fat: 0.2 g < 1%

✓ Carbs: 17.6g 6%

✓ Protein: 0.5 g 1%

✓ Cholesterol: 0 mg 0%

✓ Sodium: 9 mg < 1%

Grapefruit Rosemary Mocktails

Servings: 4 | Total time: 30 mins

Ingredients

✓ 1 cup water

✓ 1 cup Dixie Crystals granulated sugar

✓ 3 sprigs of rosemary

✓ 2 cups ruby red grapefruit juice

✓ 1/2 cup of the rosemary simple syrup

✓ 4 cups sparkling water

✓ Extra rosemary sprigs and grapefruit slices for garnish, if desired

Directions

1. Add the water and sugar to a small saucepan, over medium heat. Stir and dissolve sugar, but do not boil.

2. Once sugar has dissolved, pour the mixture into a heat safe container (I used a small mason jar) and add the rosemary sprigs. Leave rosemary in for at least an hour, then remove and discard. You can store the simple syrup in the fridge for up to ten days.

3. In a large pitcher, combine the grapefruit juice, 1/2 cup of the rosemary simple syrup, and the sparkling water. Stir to mix well, taste, and add more simple syrup, if desired.

4. Divide into glasses and garnish with rosemary and/or grapefruit slices, if desired!

Juice Cooler

"Refreshing and not-too-sweet, this cooler is easy to make. You can always use lemonade instead of cranberry juice. Or use just about any type of fruit juice you prefer."
***Servings**: 1 | **Prep**: 2 m | **Ready In**: 2 m*

Ingredients
- ✓ 6 fluid ounces cranberry juice
- ✓ 1 fluid ounce carbonated water
- ✓ 1 wedge lime

Directions
- ✓ Pour juice and carbonated water over ice. Garnish with a wedge of lime.

Nutritional Information
- ✓ Calories: 104 kcal 5%
- ✓ Fat: 0.2 g < 1%
- ✓ Carbs: 26.2g 8%
- ✓ Protein: 0 g < 1%
- ✓ Cholesterol: 0 mg 0%

✓ Sodium: 5 mg < 1%

Lime Cola

"This has been a family favorite for many years."
***Servings**: 1 | **Prep**: 1 m | **Ready In**: 1 m*

Ingredients

✓ 3 tablespoons frozen limeade concentrate, thawed
✓ 1 (12 fluid ounce) can cola-flavored carbonated beverage
✓ 1 slice lime

Directions

✓ Fill a tall glass with ice. Spoon in the limeade. Slowly pour in the cola. Garnish with a slice of lime.

Nutritional Information

✓ Calories: 299 kcal 15%
✓ Fat: 0 g < 1%
✓ Carbs: 76g 25%
✓ Protein: 0.1 g < 1%
✓ Cholesterol: 0 mg 0%
✓ Sodium: 15 mg < 1%

Lusty Lime Virgin

"Use cheap diet cola when making this drink. The sweetener makes the drink taste like it has alcohol in it, but it doesn't. Of course, you could always add some later! Delicious either way!"
***Servings**: 4 | **Prep**: 5 m | **Ready In**: 5 m*

Ingredients

✓ 1 (6 ounce) can frozen limeade concentrate

- ✓ 1 cup diet cola flavored carbonated beverage
- ✓ 1 cup orange juice
- ✓ 1 cup water
- ✓ 10 cubes ice

Directions

- ✓ Combine the limeade concentrate, carbonated beverage, orange juice, water and ice in the container of a blender. Cover, and blend until slushy. If you want to add liquor, add it last, and just blend for a few seconds more.

Nutritional Information

- ✓ Calories: 163 kcal 8%
- ✓ Fat: 0.1 g < 1%
- ✓ Carbs: 40.5g 13%
- ✓ Protein: 0.5 g < 1%
- ✓ Cholesterol: 0 mg 0%
- ✓ Sodium: 6 mg < 1%

Mango Frappe

"Pureed mango teams with orange and lime juices to make a refreshing slushy drink."

Servings: *3* | **Prep:** *5 m* | **Cook:** *5 m* | **Ready In:** *10 m*

Ingredients

- ✓ 1 mango - peeled, seeded, and cut into chunks
- ✓ 3/4 cup orange juice
- ✓ 1/4 cup lime juice
- ✓ 2 ice cubes
- ✓ 1 1/4 cups club soda

Directions

- ✓ Puree the mango in a blender until smooth. Add the orange and lime juices; blend until smooth. Add the club soda and ice cubes. Pulse the blender until the ice cubes are crushed and ingredients are blended.

Nutritional Information
- ✓ Calories: 78 kcal 4%
- ✓ Fat: 0.3 g < 1%
- ✓ Carbs: 19.9g 6%
- ✓ Protein: 0.9 g 2%
- ✓ Cholesterol: 0 mg 0%
- ✓ Sodium: 6 mg < 1%

Michigan Fizz

"Michigan cherries give this drink a tangy twist."
Servings: 1 | Prep: 1 m | Ready In: 1 m

Ingredients
- ✓ 3 tablespoons frozen cherry juice concentrate
- ✓ 1 cup ginger ale soda

Directions
- ✓ Measure concentrated cherry juice into a tall glass. Fill glass with ginger ale and stir gently.

Nutritional Information
- ✓ Calories: 189 kcal 9%
- ✓ Fat: 0 g 0%
- ✓ Carbs: 46.8g 15%
- ✓ Protein: 0 g 0%
- ✓ Cholesterol: 0 mg 0%
- ✓ Sodium: 55 mg 2%

Mock Champagne

"A good baby-shower punch that looks especially good when served with an ice ring."

*Servings: 40 | **Prep**: 1 d 15 m | **Ready In**: 1 d 15 m*

Ingredients

- ✓ 2 (2 liter) bottles ginger ale, chilled
- ✓ 1 (46 fluid ounce) can pineapple juice, chilled
- ✓ 1 (64 fluid ounce) bottle white grape juice, chilled

Directions

1. To make Ice ring: Fill a ring-shaped cake pan to 1/2 with ginger ale. Freeze until partially frozen. At this stage you can place edible flowers, or pieces of fruit around the ring. Fill pan with ginger ale and freeze until solid. Place in punch bowl just before serving.
2. In a large punch bowl, combine 1 bottle ginger ale, pineapple juice and white grape juice.

Nutritional Information

- ✓ Calories: 83 kcal 4%
- ✓ Fat: 0.1 g < 1%
- ✓ Carbs: 20.4g 7%
- ✓ Protein: 0.4 g < 1%
- ✓ Cholesterol: 0 mg 0%
- ✓ Sodium: 14 mg < 1%

Monica's Baptist Sangria

"This fresh, sweet nonalcoholic drink is beautiful in a punch bowl and will have your guests coming back for more and more!"

Servings: 12 | Prep: 10 m | Ready In: 10 m

Ingredients

- ✓ 1 (2 liter) bottle lemon-lime flavored carbonated beverage
- ✓ 1 cup instant tea powder
- ✓ 2 oranges, sliced into rounds
- ✓ 1 lemon, sliced into rounds
- ✓ 3 cups ice

Directions

- ✓ Pour the lemon-lime soda into a punch bowl, and stir in the instant iced tea. Float the orange and lemon slices in the punch, and add ice. Serve immediately.

Nutritional Information

- ✓ Calories: 86 kcal 4%
- ✓ Fat: 0 g < 1%
- ✓ Carbs: 21.6g 7%
- ✓ Protein: 0.7 g 1%
- ✓ Cholesterol: 0 mg 0%
- ✓ Sodium: 23 mg < 1%

Munkiboy's Cosmo-Not

"This refreshing non-alcoholic mocktail is cooling on a hot summer evening and festive enough for New Year's Eve."
Servings: 1 | Prep: 5 m | Ready In: 5 m

Ingredients

- ✓ 1 cup crushed ice
- ✓ 3 fluid ounces peach nectar
- ✓ 2 fluid ounces cranberry juice cocktail
- ✓ 1/2 fluid ounce grenadine syrup

- ✓ 1 fluid ounce lemon flavored carbonated beverage
- ✓ 1 twist lime peel

Directions

- ✓ Fill a shaker with ice and pour in peach nectar, cranberry juice and grenadine. Strain into a martini glass and top with lemon soda. Garnish with a twist of lime.

Nutritional Information

- ✓ Calories: 152 kcal 8%
- ✓ Fat: 0.1 g < 1%
- ✓ Carbs: 38.5g 12%
- ✓ Protein: 0.3 g < 1%
- ✓ Cholesterol: 0 mg 0%
- ✓ Sodium: 20 mg < 1%

Orange Drink

"A very simple and refreshing carbonated orange fruit drink."
Servings: *8* | **Prep:** *10 m* | **Ready In:** *10 m*

Ingredients

- ✓ 1 (12 fluid ounce) can frozen orange juice concentrate
- ✓ 2 liters ginger ale soda
- ✓ 1 orange, sliced into rounds
- ✓ 1 (4 ounce) jar maraschino cherries

Directions

1. Empty frozen orange juice into a large pitcher. VERY SLOWLY pour in the ginger ale. It is extremely important that you pour slowly because the soda will foam up and lose its carbonation if poured fast. Gently stir until all of orange juice is melted. Toss in all but 4 of the orange slices.

2. Cut reserved orange slices in half. Pour beverage into 8 glasses and garnish with half slice of orange and a cherry.

Nutritional Information

- ✓ Calories: 180 kcal 9%
- ✓ Fat: 0.1 g < 1%
- ✓ Carbs: 43.9g 14%
- ✓ Protein: 1.2 g 2%
- ✓ Cholesterol: 0 mg 0%
- ✓ Sodium: 31 mg 1%

RaSpBeRrY FiZzLeR

"This recipe, made for kids, is a fruity-good drink. Raspberry juice is blended with raspberry sherbet and carbonated water. You can try cranberry-raspberry, or apple-raspberry juice!"

Servings: 2 | **Prep**: 5 m | **Ready In**: 5 m

Ingredients

- ✓ 1 1/2 cups raspberry juice
- ✓ 3 scoops raspberry sherbet
- ✓ 1/2 cup carbonated water

Directions

- ✓ In a blender, combine raspberry juice, raspberry sherbet and carbonated water. Blend until smooth. Pour into glasses and serve.

Nutritional Information

- ✓ Calories: 90 kcal 4%
- ✓ Fat: 0 g 0%
- ✓ Carbs: 21.9g 7%
- ✓ Protein: 0.6 g 1%
- ✓ Cholesterol: 0 mg 0%
- ✓ Sodium: 7 mg < 1%

Raspberry Lime Rickey

"You can change the flavor this recipe by using any flavored syrup. For a Lemon Rickey use a lemon in place of a lime. For an Orange Rickey use an orange etc. For an alcoholic version, add a 1/2 ounce of vodka."
Servings: 1 | **Prep**: 2 m | **Ready In**: 2 m

Ingredients
- ✓ 1 lime, quartered
- ✓ 8 fluid ounces carbonated water
- ✓ 1 (1.5 fluid ounce) jigger raspberry syrup

Directions
- ✓ Fill a tall glass with ice. Squeeze each of the lime wedges into glass, and drop in. Fill glass nearly to the top with carbonated water, and top with raspberry syrup.

Nutritional Information
- ✓ Calories: 186 kcal 9%
- ✓ Fat: 0.1 g < 1%
- ✓ Carbs: 48.5g 16%
- ✓ Protein: 0.5 g < 1%
- ✓ Cholesterol: 0 mg 0%
- ✓ Sodium: 9 mg < 1%

Rhubarb Vanilla Mojito Mocktail

Rhubarb vanilla mojito mocktail recipe! A delicious, alcohol-free twist on the classic mojito cocktail made with YES Beverage's rhubarb vanilla mixer.
Servings: 1 | **Total time**: 5 mins

Ingredients

- ✓ 5-6 fresh mint leaves
- ✓ ¼ of a lime
- ✓ ¼ cup YES Artisan Beverage's rhubarb vanilla mixer
- ✓ Ice
- ✓ Sparkling water

Directions

1. In a lowball cocktail glass, muddle the mint and lime together. Add the mixer.
2. Fill glass about halfway with ice and then fill with sparkling water.
3. Give a good stir and enjoy!

Shirley Temple from 7UP

"Pretty in pink with 7UP and grenadine syrup, and naturally topped with a bright red maraschino cherry. Cheers!"
Servings: 1 | **Prep**: 5 m | **Ready In**: 5 m

Ingredients

- ✓ 8 ounces 7UP®
- ✓ 1 ounce Rose's® Grenadine Syrup
- ✓ 1 red maraschino cherry

Directions

- ✓ Plour the grenadine and lime juice into a tall glass. Pour in the cola to mix. Float a strip of lemon zest on top to garnish.

Notes

- ✓ ROSE'S and ROSE'S COCKTAIL INFUSIONS are registered trademarks of Cadbury Ireland Ltd. Used under license. 7UP, CANADA DRY and HAWAIIAN PUNCH are registered trademarks of Dr Pepper/Seven Up, Inc. (c)2012 Dr Pepper/Seven Up, Inc.

Nutritional Information

- ✓ Calories: 180 kcal 9%
- ✓ Fat: 0 g < 1%
- ✓ Carbs: 46.5g 15%
- ✓ Protein: 0 g < 1%
- ✓ Cholesterol: 0 mg 0%
- ✓ Sodium: 37 mg 1%

Strawberry-Mint Soda

"While making a pitcher of my Strawberry Mojitos, I had a request for one without any alcohol. It seemed to be a hit! You can adjust the taste by adding less or more of any ingredient. Refreshing and light, it's perfect on a hot summer day!"

Servings: *8* | **Prep**: *10 m* | **Ready In**: *10 m*

Ingredients

- ✓ 2 large limes, quartered
- ✓ 1/2 bunch mint leaves
- ✓ 7 strawberries, quartered
- ✓ 1 cup white sugar
- ✓ 3 cups carbonated water

Directions

- ✓ Squeeze the lime quarters into a sturdy glass pitcher. Toss the juiced limes into the pitcher along with the mint, strawberries, and sugar. Crush the fruits together with a muddler to release the juices from the strawberries and the oil from the mint leaves. Stir in the club soda until the sugar has dissolved. Pour into the sugared glasses over ice cubes to serve.

Nutritional Information

- ✓ Calories: 111 kcal 6%
- ✓ Fat: 0.1 g < 1%
- ✓ Carbs: 29.3g 9%
- ✓ Protein: 0.4 g < 1%
- ✓ Cholesterol: 0 mg 0%
- ✓ Sodium: 4 mg < 1%

The Arnold Palmer

"Sometimes the best things are the most simple. Nothing rings of summertime more than lemonade and iced tea. The Arnold Palmer brings them together."

*Servings: 1 | **Prep**: 5 m | **Ready In**: 5 m*

Ingredients

- ✓ 5 fluid ounces prepared lemonade
- ✓ 5 fluid ounces prepared iced tea
- ✓ 1 cup ice

Directions

- ✓ Combine lemonade and iced tea in a highball or tall glass. Add ice and stir until chilled.

Nutritional Information

- ✓ Calories: 60 kcal 3%
- ✓ Fat: 0.1 g < 1%
- ✓ Carbs: 15.6g 5%
- ✓ Protein: 0.1 g < 1%
- ✓ Cholesterol: 0 mg 0%
- ✓ Sodium: 18 mg < 1%

Tiki Cooler

"Dreaming of coladas or mojitos? Celebrating classic tiki flavors, this mocktail is bright with citrus, low on sweetness. From the first sip, imagining a beautiful beach is altogether easy."
Servings: 4 | **Prep**: 10 m | **Ready In**: 10 m

Ingredients

- ✓ Ice cubes
- ✓ 1 (6 ounce) can pineapple juice
- ✓ 6 fluid ounces coconut milk
- ✓ 3 limes, juiced
- ✓ 2 tablespoons almond-flavored syrup (such as Torani®)
- ✓ 1 cup club soda, or as needed
- ✓ 4 pinches ground nutmeg
- ✓ 4 lime wheels
- ✓ 4 sprigs fresh mint
- ✓ Cocktail umbrellas

Directions

1. Place a few ice cubes in a pitcher; add pineapple juice, coconut milk, lime juice, and almond-flavored syrup and stir until chilled. Strain mixture and pour into 4 glasses.
2. Top each glass with club soda; mocktail will foam up.
3. Dust each mocktail with nutmeg. Garnish with a lime wheel, sprig of mint, and umbrella.

Cook's Note

- ✓ Add more almond syrup or honey if you desire a sweeter drink. You may add 2 ounces of rum, if you like.

Nutritional Information

- ✓ Calories: 150 kcal 8%
- ✓ Fat: 9.7 g 15%

- ✓ Carbs: 17g 5%
- ✓ Protein: 1.3 g 3%
- ✓ Cholesterol: 0 mg 0%
- ✓ Sodium: 14 mg < 1%

Tornado Twist

"Great drink for kids and adults who don't like the bitter taste of cranberry-raspberry juice."
Servings: 2 | Prep: 1 m | Ready In: 1 m

Ingredients

- ✓ 12 fluid ounces cranberry-raspberry juice
- ✓ 1 (12 fluid ounce) can or bottle lemon-lime flavored carbonated beverage

Directions

- ✓ In a pitcher, mix cranberry-raspberry juice with lemon-lime soda. Pour over ice and serve.

Nutritional Information

- ✓ Calories: 106 kcal 5%
- ✓ Fat: 0 g 0%
- ✓ Carbs: 27.1g 9%
- ✓ Protein: 0.2 g < 1%
- ✓ Cholesterol: 0 mg 0%
- ✓ Sodium: 24 mg < 1%

Virgin Cucumber Mojito

"This is so refreshing. Cool, smooth summer drink. Delicious and super easy. The cucumber lends this drink a beautiful fresh scent and taste."
Servings: 8 | Prep: 10 m | Ready In: 10 m

Ingredients

- ✓ 1 individual packet Mojito-flavored dry beverage mix (such as Crystal Light®)
- ✓ 8 cups cold water
- ✓ 1 cucumber, peeled and sliced
- ✓ 3 cups ice cubes

Directions

- ✓ Dissolve beverage mix into cold water in a pitcher; add cucumber slices and ice cubes.

Nutritional Information

- ✓ Calories: 6 kcal < 1%
- ✓ Fat: 0 g < 1%
- ✓ Carbs: 0.6g < 1%
- ✓ Protein: 0.1 g < 1%
- ✓ Cholesterol: 0 mg 0%
- ✓ Sodium: 10 mg < 1%

Virgin Pina Colada

"A yummy, easy to make tropical fruit drink recipe using everyday ingredients! Great for those hot days by the pool!"
***Servings:** 2 | **Prep:** 2 m | **Ready In:** 2 m*

Ingredients

- ✓ 1 cup ice
- ✓ 1 1/4 cups pineapple juice
- ✓ 1/2 cup milk
- ✓ 1/2 cup heavy cream
- ✓ 2 tablespoons white sugar

Directions

- ✓ In an electric blender, blend ice, pineapple juice, milk, cream, and sugar. Blend until smooth.

Nutritional Information

- ✓ Calories: 367 kcal 18%
- ✓ Fat: 23.4 g 36%
- ✓ Carbs: 37.1g 12%
- ✓ Protein: 3.8 g 8%
- ✓ Cholesterol: 86 mg 29%
- ✓ Sodium: 54 mg 2%

Virgin Strawberry Daiquiri

"I love to drink these when I'm out on the town."
***Servings**: 1 | **Prep**: 2 m | **Ready In**: 2 m*

Ingredients

- ✓ 3 1/2 ounces frozen strawberries
- ✓ 1/8 cup ice
- ✓ 1/2 fluid ounce sweet and sour mix
- ✓ 1 dash grenadine syrup

Directions

- ✓ Place strawberries, ice cubes, sweet and sour mix and grenadine in a blender. Blend until smooth. Add more ice or less depending on your taste.

Nutritional Information

- ✓ Calories: 67 kcal 3%
- ✓ Fat: 0.1 g < 1%
- ✓ Carbs: 15.6g 5%
- ✓ Protein: 0.4 g < 1%
- ✓ Cholesterol: 0 mg 0%
- ✓ Sodium: 3 mg < 1%

Watermelon Fizz

"Mouth-watering nutritious mocktail with the power of coconut water and watermelon. Garnish with an orange twist, watermelon wedge, and grapes with two blending straws."
***Servings**: 4 | **Prep**: 5 m | **Ready In**: 5 m*

Ingredients
- ✓ 1 cup coconut water
- ✓ 1/2 cup watermelon puree
- ✓ 1 teaspoon stevia
- ✓ 1/2 cup ice cubes, or as desired

Directions
1. Blend coconut water, watermelon, and stevia together in a blender until smooth.
2. Fill a cocktail shaker with ice; add watermelon mixture. Cover shaker and shake until chilled; pour into a poco grande glass.

Nutritional Information
- ✓ Calories: 82 kcal 4%
- ✓ Fat: 0.6 g < 1%
- ✓ Carbs: 20.1g 6%
- ✓ Protein: 2.4 g 5%
- ✓ Cholesterol: 0 mg 0%
- ✓ Sodium: 255 mg 10

Five: Non-alcoholic Punch

* * *

Punch is the term for a wide assortment of drinks, both non-alcoholic and alcoholic, generally containing fruit or fruit juice. The drink was introduced from India to the United Kingdom in the early seventeenth century, and from there its use spread to other countries. Punch is typically served at parties in large, wide bowls, known as punch bowls. Sangria is a kind of punch.

*_Wikipedia_*

Candie's SIMPLY Great Punch

"Believe it or not, the party punch that people flip over is the easiest to make! Quit fooling with all those measurements and come on over to the easy side of the street! By the way, the French vanilla that always seems to taste the best in this punch are the cheap off-brands. Sounds like a line, but it's true!"

***Servings:** 80 | **Prep:** 2 m | **Ready In:** 2 m*

Ingredients

- ✓ 2 (46 fluid ounce) cans fruit punch
- ✓ 1 (2 liter) bottle lemon-lime flavored carbonated beverage
- ✓ 1/2 gallon French vanilla ice cream

Directions

- ✓ Pour chilled punch and soda into punch bowl. Scoop out entire half-gallon of ice cream, and carefully slide into punch.

Nutritional Information

- ✓ Calories: 80 kcal 4%
- ✓ Fat: 3.6 g 6%
- ✓ Carbs: 10.8g 3%
- ✓ Protein: 1 g 2%
- ✓ Cholesterol: 24 mg 8%
- ✓ Sodium: 32 mg 1%

Holiday Cranberry Punch

"My mother made this drink every Thanksgiving and Christmas. It is one family tradition I can't live without."

*Servings: 7 | **Prep**: 10 m | **Ready In**: 10 m*

Ingredients

- ✓ 1 (16 ounce) can jellied cranberry sauce
- ✓ 3/4 cup orange juice
- ✓ 1/4 cup lemon juice
- ✓ 2 cups ice, or as needed
- ✓ 3 1/2 cups chilled ginger ale

Directions

1. Blend cranberry sauce in a blender until smooth; add orange juice and lemon juice and blend again until smooth.
2. Combine cranberry mixture and ice in a pitcher. Slowly pour ginger ale into cranberry mixture and gently stir to combine.

Nutritional Information

- ✓ Calories: 154 kcal 8%
- ✓ Fat: 0.1 g < 1%
- ✓ Carbs: 39.1g 13%
- ✓ Protein: 0.3 g < 1%
- ✓ Cholesterol: 0 mg 0%
- ✓ Sodium: 36 mg 1%

Holiday Red Punch

"A delicious Christmas red punch for everyone--children love it."
*Servings: 34 | **Prep**: 10 m | **Ready In**: 10 m*

Ingredients

- ✓ 4 cups apple juice
- ✓ 1 (46 fluid ounce) can fruit punch
- ✓ 1 (6 ounce) can frozen lemonade concentrate, thawed

- ✓ 1 (6 ounce) can frozen pink lemonade concentrate, thawed
- ✓ 18 fluid ounces water
- ✓ 1 tablespoon red food coloring

Directions

- ✓ In a large punch bowl combine apple juice, fruit punch, lemonade concentrate, pink lemonade concentrate, water and food coloring. Mix well.

Nutritional Information

- ✓ Calories: 55 kcal 3%
- ✓ Fat: 0.1 g < 1%
- ✓ Carbs: 14g 5%
- ✓ Protein: 0.1 g < 1%
- ✓ Cholesterol: 0 mg 0%
- ✓ Sodium: 16 mg < 1%

Honey Limeade

"A refreshing drink on a hot day. Serve over ice."
***Servings**: 6 | **Prep**: 15 m | **Ready In**: 15 m*

Ingredients

- ✓ 1 cup lime juice
- ✓ 5 cups water
- ✓ 2/3 cup white sugar
- ✓ 2 tablespoons honey

Directions

- ✓ In a pitcher, combine lime juice, water, sugar and honey. Stir until sugar is dissolved. Chill in refrigerator.

Nutritional Information

- ✓ Calories: 118 kcal 6%
- ✓ Fat: 0 g < 1%

✓ Carbs: 31.4g 10%
✓ Protein: 0.2 g < 1%
✓ Cholesterol: 0 mg 0%
✓ Sodium: 1 mg < 1%

Hot Cider Punch

"A spicy blend of apple, pineapple, and cranberry juices, this hot punch seasoned with cinnamon sticks, cloves, and allspice makes a perfect holiday beverage."
Servings: 15 | **Prep**: 5 m | **Cook**: 10 m | **Ready In**: 15 m

Ingredients
✓ 3 cups apple juice
✓ 2 1/2 cups unsweetened pineapple juice
✓ 2 cups cranberry juice
✓ 1/4 cup brown sugar
✓ 2 cinnamon sticks
✓ 2 teaspoons whole cloves
✓ 2 teaspoons ground allspice

Directions
✓ Stir the apple juice, pineapple juice, and cranberry juice together with the brown sugar in a large pan. Place the cinnamon sticks, cloves, and ground allspice into a large teaball or cheesecloth bag. Place the spice bag into the pan with the juice mixture. Heat the juice mixture over medium-high heat about 10 minutes. Serve hot.

Nutritional Information
✓ Calories: 83 kcal 4%
✓ Fat: 0.2 g < 1%
✓ Carbs: 20.5g 7%
✓ Protein: 0.3 g < 1%

✓ Cholesterol: 0 mg 0%

✓ Sodium: 5 mg < 1%

Hot Cranberry Citrus Punch

"This tart punch warms you on a cold winter's night. I always serve it for Christmas Eve dinner. The longer it cooks, the better it tastes!"

Servings: *20* | **Prep:** *10 m* | **Cook:** *6 h* | **Ready In:** *6 h 10 m*

Ingredients

✓ 2 quarts cranberry juice cocktail

✓ 3 cups orange juice

✓ 1/4 cup white sugar

✓ 1/4 cup brown sugar

✓ 2 tablespoons fresh lemon juice

✓ 1 pinch salt

✓ 2 (3 inch) cinnamon sticks

Directions

✓ In a 4 quart or larger slow cooker, combine the cranberry juice, orange juice, white sugar, brown sugar, lemon juice, salt and cinnamon sticks. Stir to dissolve sugar. Cook on High for 4 to 6 hours. Turn heat to Low and keep warm for serving.

Easy Cleanup

✓ Try using a liner in your slow cooker for easier cleanup.

Nutritional Information

✓ Calories: 93 kcal 5%

✓ Fat: 0.2 g < 1%

✓ Carbs: 23.2g 7%

✓ Protein: 0.3 g < 1%

✓ Cholesterol: 0 mg 0%

✓ Sodium: 11 mg < 1%

Incredible Punch

"Absolutely the best punch! A hit at showers, teas and kids' birthday parties. It's made with cran-raspberry juice, ginger ale and pina colada mixer and has a beautiful pink color!."
Servings*: 50 | **Prep***: 10 m | ***Ready In****: 10 m*

Ingredients
- ✓ 2 (46 fluid ounce) bottles cranberry-raspberry juice
- ✓ 1 (32 fluid ounce) bottle pina colada mix
- ✓ 2 liters raspberry ginger ale soda

Directions
1. In a large plastic container, combine cranberry-raspberry juice with the pina colada mix. Freeze overnight.
2. Remove from freezer 30 minutes prior to serving. To serve place frozen slush in punch bowl and slowly add raspberry ginger ale.

Nutritional Information
- ✓ Calories: 44 kcal 2%
- ✓ Fat: 0.4 g < 1%
- ✓ Carbs: 10.2g 3%
- ✓ Protein: 0.1 g < 1%
- ✓ Cholesterol: 0 mg 0%
- ✓ Sodium: 7 mg < 1%

Kelly's Super Simple Shower Punch

"This is a fabulously simple and delicious punch. It has only 2 ingredients!"
Servings*: 16 | **Prep***: 5 m | ***Ready In****: 5 m*

Ingredients

- ✓ 1 pint raspberry sorbet
- ✓ 1 (2 liter) bottle lemon-lime soda

Directions

- ✓ Spoon the sorbet into the bottom of a punch bowl. Slowly pour the soda over the sorbet. Use the back of a spoon to soften the sorbet until combined.

Nutritional Information

- ✓ Calories: 84 kcal 4%
- ✓ Fat: 0 g 0%
- ✓ Carbs: 21.5g 7%
- ✓ Protein: 0 g 0%
- ✓ Cholesterol: 0 mg 0%
- ✓ Sodium: 14 mg < 1%

Kiddie Holiday Juice

"This is really great for the holidays and kids just love it even when they hate cranberry juice!"

***Servings**: 15 | **Prep**: 5 m | **Ready In**: 5 m*

Ingredients

- ✓ 1 (64 fluid ounce) bottle cranberry juice
- ✓ 4 liters lemon-lime flavored carbonated beverage
- ✓ 3 oranges, sliced into rounds
- ✓ 8 cups crushed ice

Directions

- ✓ In a large punch bowl, combine cranberry juice and orange slices. Pour in the lemon lime soda and crushed ice. Serve immediately.

Nutritional Information

- ✓ Calories: 136 kcal 7%

- ✓ Fat: 0.1 g < 1%
- ✓ Carbs: 34.9g 11%
- ✓ Protein: 0.2 g < 1%
- ✓ Cholesterol: 0 mg 0%
- ✓ Sodium: 24 mg < 1%

Kool Ade Punch

"Makes a delicious drink and you can also float ice cream or sherbet on top."

Servings: 24 | Prep: 10 m | Ready In: 10 m

Ingredients

- ✓ 1 (4.6 ounce) package cherry flavored sweetened soft drink mix
- ✓ 1 (46 fluid ounce) can unsweetened pineapple juice
- ✓ 1 liter lemon-lime flavored carbonated beverage
- ✓ 1 (6 ounce) can frozen orange juice concentrate, thawed
- ✓ 1 (6 ounce) can frozen lemonade concentrate, thawed

Directions

- ✓ In a punch bowl prepare drink mix according to package instructions. Stir in pineapple juice and lemon-lime soda. Mix in the concentrated orange juice and lemonade. Refrigerate until ready to serve.

Nutritional Information

- ✓ Calories: 96 kcal 5%
- ✓ Fat: 0.1 g < 1%
- ✓ Carbs: 24.4g 8%
- ✓ Protein: 0.4 g < 1%
- ✓ Cholesterol: 0 mg 0%
- ✓ Sodium: 6 mg < 1%

Lemonade

"A cool refreshing summer drink that can be made at any time you have lemons... or limes!"
Servings: *32 |* ***Prep:*** *10 m |* ***Ready In:*** *10 m*

Ingredients
- ✓ 4 lemons, juiced
- ✓ 1 quart water
- ✓ 1/2 cup white sugar

Directions
- ✓ In a 2 quart pitcher, combine the lemon juice, water and sugar. Stir until sugar is dissolved. Chill in refrigerator.

Nutritional Information
- ✓ Calories: 86 kcal 4%
- ✓ Fat: 0 g 0%
- ✓ Carbs: 23.1g 7%
- ✓ Protein: 0.1 g < 1%
- ✓ Cholesterol: 0 mg 0%
- ✓ Sodium: 6 mg < 1%

Lime Sherbet Punch

"A holiday favorite that everyone looks for year after year. You'll learn to buy the lime sherbet in advance since the stores sell out around the holidays."
Servings: *18 |* ***Prep:*** *10 m |* ***Ready In:*** *10 m*

Ingredients
- ✓ 2 quarts lime sherbet
- ✓ 2 (2 liter) bottles ginger ale
- ✓ 1 (46 fluid ounce) can pineapple juice

- ✓ 1 (4 ounce) jar maraschino cherries, drained
- ✓ 1 lemon, sliced
- ✓ 1 lime, sliced

Directions

1. Scoop lime sherbet into a punch bowl; pour in ginger ale and pineapple juice. Stir well.
2. Stir in maraschino cherries and float lemon and lime slices in the punch.

Nutritional Information

- ✓ Calories: 246 kcal 12%
- ✓ Fat: 1.9 g 3%
- ✓ Carbs: 57.8g 19%
- ✓ Protein: 1.3 g 3%
- ✓ Cholesterol: 5 mg 2%
- ✓ Sodium: 68 mg 3%

Limeade

"A delicious and refreshing drink made with limes. Serve over ice on a hot day."

Servings: 8 | **Prep**: 10 m | **Ready In**: 10 m

Ingredients

- ✓ 3 limes
- ✓ 2/3 cup white sugar
- ✓ 2 quarts cold water

Directions

- ✓ Cut limes in half and squeeze lime juice into a 2 quart pitcher. Add sugar and stir until dissolved. Fill pitcher with cold water, stir and chill in refrigerator.

Nutritional Information

- ✓ Calories: 72 kcal 4%

✓ Fat: 0.1 g < 1%
✓ Carbs: 19.3g 6%
✓ Protein: 0.2 g < 1%
✓ Cholesterol: 0 mg 0%
✓ Sodium: 8 mg < 1%

Lime-Pineapple Delight

"This punch is a special occasion family punch. Great to serve on Christmas, Thanksgiving and any time."
***Servings**: 10 | **Prep**: 5 m | **Ready In**: 10 m*

Ingredients

✓ 8 cups crushed ice
✓ 3 (0.13 ounce) packages unsweetened lemon-lime flavored drink mix
✓ 3 cups white sugar
✓ 1 (46 fluid ounce) can pineapple juice, chilled
✓ 1/2 gallon lime sherbet
✓ 3 liters lemon-lime flavored carbonated beverage

Directions

✓ Fill punch bowl 1/2 full with ice. Add drink mix, sugar and pineapple juice. Sir to dissolve. Place lime sherbet in punch bowl. Pour in the carbonated beverage. Gently stir and then serve in chilled glasses.

Nutritional Information

✓ Calories: 634 kcal 32%
✓ Fat: 3.3 g 5%
✓ Carbs: 154.6g 50%
✓ Protein: 2.2 g 4%
✓ Cholesterol: 9 mg 3%
✓ Sodium: 114 mg 5%

Luau Punch

"This slushy fruit punch has been used for years by my family at birthday parties, summer gatherings and now my children ask for it at breakfast...it is our favorite punch. We make it in an empty gallon milk jug."

***Servings**: 10 | **Prep**: 10 m | **Ready In**: 10 m*

Ingredients

- ✓ 1 (46 fluid ounce) can pineapple juice
- ✓ 1 (6 ounce) can frozen orange juice concentrate, thawed
- ✓ 2 liters lemon-lime flavored carbonated beverage

Directions

1. In an empty gallon milk jug or pitcher, pour pineapple juice and orange juice concentrate. Shake to mix and pour in the lemon-lime soda. You may need to let the fizz settle and then return to pouring. This will fill up the gallon. Freeze overnight.
2. Let the punch start to thaw 2 hours before serving. Serve slushy.

Nutritional Information

- ✓ Calories: 182 kcal 9%
- ✓ Fat: 0.2 g < 1%
- ✓ Carbs: 45.3g 15%
- ✓ Protein: 1 g 2%
- ✓ Cholesterol: 0 mg 0%
- ✓ Sodium: 24 mg < 1%

Luscious Slush Punch

"This is without a doubt the best punch I've ever had! Makes enough for 2 punch bowls. This is our Christmas Eve punch tradition, and there is never a drop left!"

***Servings**: 50 | **Prep**: 15 m | **Cook**: 5 m | **Ready In**: 8 h 20 m*

Ingredients

- ✓ 2 1/2 cups white sugar
- ✓ 6 cups water
- ✓ 2 (3 ounce) packages strawberry flavored Jell-O® mix
- ✓ 1 (46 fluid ounce) can pineapple juice
- ✓ 2/3 cup lemon juice
- ✓ 1 quart orange juice
- ✓ 2 (2 liter) bottles lemon-lime flavored carbonated beverage

Directions

1. Bring the sugar, water, and strawberry flavored gelatin to a boil in a large saucepan; boil for 3 minutes. Stir in the pineapple juice, lemon juice, and orange juice. Divide mixture into 2 separate containers and freeze.

2. Combine the contents of 1 container with 1 bottle of the lemon-lime flavored carbonated beverage in a punch bowl; stir until slushy. Repeat with remaining portions as needed.

Nutritional Information

- ✓ Calories: 108 kcal 5%
- ✓ Fat: 0.1 g < 1%
- ✓ Carbs: 27.4g 9%
- ✓ Protein: 0.6 g 1%
- ✓ Cholesterol: 0 mg 0%
- ✓ Sodium: 25 mg < 1%

Melon Chiller

"This cantaloupe drink is easy to make and very refreshing, especially on a hot, sunny day. It's a real crowd-pleaser too!"
***Servings**: 10 | **Prep**: 20 m | **Ready In**: 20 m*

Ingredients
- ✓ 1 cantaloupe, halved and seeded
- ✓ 1 gallon water
- ✓ 2 cups white sugar
- ✓ Ice cubes, as needed

Directions
- ✓ Scrape the cantaloupe meat lengthwise with a spoon or a melon baller and place in a punch bowl; add the water and sugar. Mix thoroughly until all the sugar is dissolved. Chill with the addition of plenty of ice cubes.

Nutritional Information
- ✓ Calories: 174 kcal 9%
- ✓ Fat: 0.1 g < 1%
- ✓ Carbs: 44.5g 14%
- ✓ Protein: 0.5 g < 1%
- ✓ Cholesterol: 0 mg 0%
- ✓ Sodium: 23 mg < 1%

Mint Tea Punch

"Tea, mint, sugar, orange and lemon juices make this a quick and easy, refreshingly delicious drink on a hot summer's day, given to me by a true Southern lady. Goes great with Cajun or spicy foods too. Every time I serve this someone asks me for the recipe!"
***Servings**: 10 | **Prep**: 10 m | **Ready In**: 10 m*

Ingredients

- ✓ 3 cups boiling water
- ✓ 12 sprigs fresh mint
- ✓ 4 tea bags
- ✓ 1 cup white sugar
- ✓ 1 cup orange juice
- ✓ 1/4 cup lemon juice
- ✓ 5 cups cold water
- ✓ 3 orange slices for garnish (optional)
- ✓ 3 lemon slices for garnish (optional)

Directions

- ✓ Place the tea bags and mint sprigs into a large pitcher. Pour boiling water over them, and allow to steep for about 8 minutes. Remove and discard the tea bags and mint leaves, squeezing out excess liquid. Stir in sugar until dissolved, then stir in the orange juice and lemon juice. Pour in the cold water. Serve over ice cubes, garnished with orange or lemon slices.

Nutritional Information

- ✓ Calories: 94 kcal 5%
- ✓ Fat: 0.1 g < 1%
- ✓ Carbs: 24.2g 8%
- ✓ Protein: 0.4 g < 1%
- ✓ Cholesterol: 0 mg 0%
- ✓ Sodium: 6 mg < 1%

Mock Pink Champagne

"Lots of fruit juice and color make this sparkly, bubbly punch a real crowd pleaser."

Servings: 24 | **Prep:** 10 m | **Ready In:** 10 m

Ingredients

- ✓ 1/2 cup sugar
- ✓ 1 1/2 cups water
- ✓ 1/2 cup orange juice
- ✓ 2 cups cranberry juice
- ✓ 1 cup pineapple juice
- ✓ 4 cups 7UP®

Directions

1. Combine all ingredients.
2. Serve in champagne flutes.

Nutritional Information

- ✓ Calories: 51 kcal 3%
- ✓ Fat: 0 g < 1%
- ✓ Carbs: 13g 4%
- ✓ Protein: 0.1 g < 1%
- ✓ Cholesterol: 0 mg 0%
- ✓ Sodium: 6 mg < 1%

Mormon Champagne

"A yummy, simple drink with white grape juice and grapefruit soda. Great for parties, showers, or just for fun!!!"

Servings: *16 |* ***Prep:*** *5 m |* ***Ready In:*** *5 m*

Ingredients

- ✓ 1 (2 liter) bottle grapefruit flavored soda (such as Fresca®), chilled
- ✓ 1 (64 fluid ounce) bottle white grape juice, chilled

Directions

- ✓ Mix together the grapefruit soda and grape juice in a large bowl. Serve in champagne or punch glasses.

Nutritional Information

- ✓ Calories: 127 kcal 6%
- ✓ Fat: 0.1 g < 1%
- ✓ Carbs: 31.5g 10%
- ✓ Protein: 0.7 g 1%
- ✓ Cholesterol: 0 mg 0%
- ✓ Sodium: 7 mg < 1%

New York State Special Milk Punch

"This is a quick and easy recipe that's great for the summer."
Servings: *10 |* **Prep:** *15 m |* **Ready In:** *20 m*

Ingredients

- ✓ 1 1/2 quarts vanilla ice cream, softened
- ✓ 3 (46 fluid ounce) cans pineapple juice, chilled
- ✓ 1/2 cup orange juice
- ✓ 1 tablespoon lemon juice
- ✓ 1 quart cold milk

Directions

- ✓ In a punch bowl, combine ice cream, pineapple juice, orange juice, lemon juice and milk. Stir until ingredients are blended.

Nutritional Information

- ✓ Calories: 429 kcal 21%
- ✓ Fat: 11.1 g 17%
- ✓ Carbs: 76.9g 25%
- ✓ Protein: 7.5 g 15%
- ✓ Cholesterol: 43 mg 14%
- ✓ Sodium: 112 mg 4%

Nonalco Punch

"I have great demand for this recipe at all our church functions and showers. It's great with cranberry ginger ale."
Servings: 24 | **Prep**: 20 m | **Ready In**: 20 m

Ingredients
- ✓ 4 cups cranberry juice
- ✓ 4 cups pineapple juice
- ✓ 1 1/2 cups white sugar
- ✓ 1 teaspoon almond extract
- ✓ 1 liter ginger ale soda

Directions
- ✓ In a large punch bowl, combine cranberry juice, pineapple juice and sugar. Stir until sugar is dissolved. Add almond extract and pour in the ginger ale.

Nutritional Information
- ✓ Calories: 108 kcal 5%
- ✓ Fat: 0.1 g < 1%
- ✓ Carbs: 27.1g 9%
- ✓ Protein: 0.2 g < 1%
- ✓ Cholesterol: 0 mg 0%
- ✓ Sodium: 7 mg < 1%

Non-Alcoholic New Years Eve Punch

"This recipe is great for kids or designated drivers. It is great for all occasions, but it is really popular on New Year's. Serve into ice-filled glasses."
Servings: 15 | **Prep**: 5 m | **Ready In**: 5 m

Ingredients

- ✓ 3 1/2 liters ginger ale
- ✓ 2 quarts orange juice
- ✓ 2 oranges, sliced into rounds
- ✓ 20 maraschino cherries

Directions

- ✓ In a large punch bowl mix ginger ale and orange juice. Place sliced oranges on top of punch and arrange the cherries on top of the orange slices.

Nutritional Information

- ✓ Calories: 161 kcal 8%
- ✓ Fat: 0.3 g < 1%
- ✓ Carbs: 38.8g 13%
- ✓ Protein: 1.1 g 2%
- ✓ Cholesterol: 0 mg 0%
- ✓ Sodium: 29 mg 1%

Old-Fashioned Pink Lemonade

"This is a wonderfully refreshing drink. Serve in pitchers garnished with mint leaves and orange or lemon slices."
Servings: 12 | **Prep**: 10 m | **Ready In**: 10 m

Ingredients

- ✓ 2 cups white sugar
- ✓ 9 cups water
- ✓ 2 cups fresh lemon juice
- ✓ 1 cup cranberry juice, chilled

Directions

- ✓ In large pitcher combine sugar, water, lemon juice and cranberry juice. Stir to dissolve sugar. Serve over ice.

Nutritional Information
- ✓ Calories: 151 kcal 8%
- ✓ Fat: 0 g < 1%
- ✓ Carbs: 39.7g 13%
- ✓ Protein: 0.2 g < 1%
- ✓ Cholesterol: 0 mg 0%
- ✓ Sodium: < 1 mg < 1%

Orange Cream Milk Punch

"Excellent for kids parties!"
***Servings**: 24 | **Prep**: 10 m | **Ready In**: 10 m*

Ingredients
- ✓ 1 quart vanilla ice cream
- ✓ 2 pints orange sherbet
- ✓ 1 (16 ounce) can lemon-lime flavored carbonated beverage
- ✓ 1 quart cold milk

Directions
- ✓ Place the ice cream and sherbet in a punch bowl. Pour in the milk and lemon-lime soda. Stir gently and serve immediately.

Nutritional Information
- ✓ Calories: 73 kcal 4%
- ✓ Fat: 3.2 g 5%
- ✓ Carbs: 9.2g 3%
- ✓ Protein: 2.1 g 4%
- ✓ Cholesterol: 13 mg 4%
- ✓ Sodium: 37 mg 1%

Orange Dream Punch

"This is the easiest punch recipe ever. It was a big hit at my sister's bridal shower."
Servings: *30 |* ***Prep:*** *15 m |* ***Ready In:*** *15 m*

Ingredients
- ✓ 1/2 gallon orange sherbet
- ✓ 1 (6 ounce) can frozen orange juice concentrate
- ✓ 1 (2 liter) bottle ginger ale

Directions
- ✓ Place sherbet and frozen orange juice concentrate in a punch bowl. Allow to thaw for 10 to 15 minutes. Stir in ginger ale.

Nutritional Information
- ✓ Calories: 34 kcal 2%
- ✓ Fat: 0 g < 1%
- ✓ Carbs: 8.4g 3%
- ✓ Protein: 0.2 g < 1%
- ✓ Cholesterol: 0 mg 0%
- ✓ Sodium: 8 mg < 1%

Orange Summer Cooler

"This is a great Fourth of July people pleaser. Or anytime, especially if you live under the hot Southern summer sun. Feel free to experiment with different flavors of sherbet!"
Servings: *6 |* ***Prep:*** *10 m |* ***Ready In:*** *10 m*

Ingredients
- ✓ 2 cups orange juice
- ✓ 2 cups cold water

- ✓ 2 cups orange sherbet
- ✓ 1 teaspoon vanilla extract
- ✓ 1 cup confectioners' sugar
- ✓ 3 cups crushed ice

Directions

- ✓ In a blender, blend the orange juice, water, orange sherbet, vanilla, confectioners' sugar, and ice until smooth.

Nutritional Information

- ✓ Calories: 189 kcal 9%
- ✓ Fat: 1.2 g 2%
- ✓ Carbs: 44.5g 14%
- ✓ Protein: 1.1 g 2%
- ✓ Cholesterol: 3 mg < 1%
- ✓ Sodium: 28 mg 1%

Peppermint Punch

"This wonderfully unusual punch is my husband's grandmother's recipe. I normally don't like punch...but the first time I tried this punch I couldn't get enough! Kids love it, too. Makes a nice holiday and shower punch."

Servings: 24 | **Prep**: 5 m | **Ready In**: 5 m

Ingredients

- ✓ 1 quart peppermint ice cream
- ✓ 1 cup cold milk
- ✓ 2 liters ginger ale, chilled

Directions

- ✓ Place ice cream in a punch bowl, and allow to soften slightly. Blend in milk and ginger ale. Stir until frothy. Serve at once, or keep chilled until ready to serve.

Nutritional Information

- ✓ Calories: 137 kcal 7%
- ✓ Fat: 7.1 g 11%
- ✓ Carbs: 16.2g 5%
- ✓ Protein: 2.1 g 4%
- ✓ Cholesterol: 34 mg 11%
- ✓ Sodium: 37 mg 1%

Perfect Party Punch

"This punch is made at all our family gatherings. You can add vodka to taste for an adult party."
Servings: *30* | **Prep:** *10 m* | **Ready In:** *10 m*

Ingredients

- ✓ 1 (64 fluid ounce) bottle fruit punch
- ✓ 2 (15 ounce) cans pineapple chunks
- ✓ 1 pint strawberries, hulled and sliced
- ✓ 2 bananas, sliced
- ✓ 2 pints fruit flavored sherbet
- ✓ 1 (2 liter) bottle lemon-lime flavored carbonated beverage

Directions

- ✓ In a large punch bowl, pour fruit punch. Add pineapple chunks, strawberries and bananas. Slide in the sherbet and slowly pour in the lemon-lime soda.

Nutritional Information

- ✓ Calories: 105 kcal 5%
- ✓ Fat: 0.1 g < 1%
- ✓ Carbs: 26.9g 9%
- ✓ Protein: 0.6 g 1%
- ✓ Cholesterol: 0 mg 0%

✓ Sodium: 33 mg 1%

Pink Lady Punch

"Very good punch! Good for parties and other festivities. Best served cold...obviously."
***Servings**: 16 | **Prep**: 10 m | **Ready In**: 10 m*

Ingredients
- ✓ 1 quart ginger ale, chilled
- ✓ 4 cups cranberry juice cocktail, chilled
- ✓ 4 cups pineapple juice, chilled
- ✓ 1 cup white sugar

Directions
- ✓ Mix ginger ale, cranberry juice, and pineapple juice together in a punch bowl; stir in sugar until dissolved.

Nutritional Information
- ✓ Calories: 137 kcal 7%
- ✓ Fat: 0.1 g < 1%
- ✓ Carbs: 34.4g 11%
- ✓ Protein: 0.2 g < 1%
- ✓ Cholesterol: 0 mg 0%
- ✓ Sodium: 10 mg < 1%

Ponche de Frutas (Fruit Punch)

"This Mexican punch is quite flavorful. With or without the fruit floating in your glass, it makes for a nice beverage."
***Servings**: 20 | **Prep**: 20 m | **Ready In**: 20 m*

Ingredients

- ✓ 3 oranges, juiced
- ✓ 3 lemons, juiced
- ✓ 1/2 pound seedless green grapes, halved
- ✓ 1/2 pound plums, pitted and chopped into small bite-size pieces
- ✓ 1 fresh pineapple - peeled, cored and chopped into small bite-size pieces
- ✓ 1 cup white sugar
- ✓ 4 cups strong brewed black tea, chilled
- ✓ 4 cups crushed ice

Directions

- ✓ In a large punch bowl, combine orange juice, lemon juice, grapes, plums and pineapple. Stir in sugar. Pour in tea and crushed ice.

Nutritional Information

- ✓ Calories: 79 kcal 4%
- ✓ Fat: 0.2 g < 1%
- ✓ Carbs: 21.2g 7%
- ✓ Protein: 0.7 g 1%
- ✓ Cholesterol: 0 mg 0%
- ✓ Sodium: 4 mg < 1%

Punch

"Get Fruity! This is an simple to make and very tasty punch. "
***Servings:** 50 | **Prep:** 5 m | **Ready In:** 5 m*

Ingredients

- ✓ 32 fluid ounces cranberry juice
- ✓ 32 fluid ounces lemonade
- ✓ 32 fluid ounces orange juice

- ✓ 32 fluid ounces pineapple juice
- ✓ 32 fluid ounces ginger ale

Directions

- ✓ Chill all of the juices and ginger ale. Combine them in a large punch bowl when ready to serve.

Nutritional Information

- ✓ Calories: 47 kcal 2%
- ✓ Fat: 0.1 g < 1%
- ✓ Carbs: 11.5g 4%
- ✓ Protein: 0.2 g < 1%
- ✓ Cholesterol: 0 mg 0%
- ✓ Sodium: 5 mg < 1%

Quenching Creamy Raspberry Punch

"A delicious raspberry punch that goes great with chocolate. Use either vanilla ice cream or raspberry sherbet."
***Servings**: 20 | **Prep**: 10 m | **Ready In**: 10 m*

Ingredients

- ✓ 2 (64 fluid ounce) bottles raspberry cream soda, chilled
- ✓ 1 (12 fluid ounce) can frozen concentrated raspberry juice
- ✓ 1/2 gallon vanilla ice cream

Directions

- ✓ In large punch bowl combine both bottles of raspberry cream soda and raspberry juice concentrate. Stir until concentrate is dissolved. Carefully add ice cream. Stir briefly. Best served chilled.

Nutritional Information

- ✓ Calories: 244 kcal 12%

✓ Fat: 5.8 g 9%

✓ Carbs: 46.6g 15%

✓ Protein: 2.2 g 4%

✓ Cholesterol: 23 mg 8%

✓ Sodium: 57 mg 2%

Quick and Easy Witches' Brew

"A quick-and-easy Halloween punch that kids adore at parties and church events. It also has very little sugar and is made with real fruit, so you parents only have to worry about their candy intake!"

Servings: 10 | *Prep*: 10 m | *Ready In*: 10 m

Ingredients

✓ 1 quart lime sherbet

✓ 1 (2 liter) bottle diet lemon-lime carbonated beverage

Directions

1. Place sherbet in a microwave-safe bowl; heat in microwave until slightly melted, about 10 seconds.

2. Stir lemon-lime beverage, about 1/2 cup at a time, into sherbet until punch is the texture of a milkshake. Pour punch into a large punch bowl. Slowly stir the remaining lemon-lime beverage into punch.

Nutritional Information

✓ Calories: 110 kcal 5%

✓ Fat: 1.6 g 2%

✓ Carbs: 23.7g 8%

✓ Protein: 0.9 g 2%

✓ Cholesterol: 5 mg 2%

✓ Sodium: 36 mg 1%

Red Slush Punch

"This Red Slush Punch is a party MUST! It is sooo delicious, I make it for almost every occasion!"

***Servings**: 64 | **Prep**: 15 m | **Ready In**: 3 h 15 m*

Ingredients

- ✓ 3 (3 ounce) packages strawberry flavored Jell-O® mix
- ✓ 9 cups boiling water
- ✓ 4 cups sugar
- ✓ 9 cups water
- ✓ 2 (46 fluid ounce) cans pineapple juice
- ✓ 2 cups lemon juice
- ✓ 4 (2 liter) bottles ginger ale

Directions

1. In a large bowl, whisk together the strawberry gelatin mix and 9 cups of boiling water. Set aside. In a large pot, bring the remaining 9 cups of water to a boil. Stir in the sugar until dissolved. Pour the sugar water into the gelatin water, then stir in the pineapple juice and lemon juice, mixing well. Pour into four 1-gallon size resealable freezer bags, or pretty Bundt pans to freeze.

2. To make punch, place one of the frozen portions into a punch bowl, and pour 1 bottle of ginger ale over.

Nutritional Information

- ✓ Calories: 130 kcal 7%
- ✓ Fat: 0.1 g < 1%
- ✓ Carbs: 32.6g 11%
- ✓ Protein: 0.5 g 1%
- ✓ Cholesterol: 0 mg 0%
- ✓ Sodium: 34 mg 1%

Sherbet Shower Surprise

"This punch is always great for Bridal and Baby showers! You just can't get enough! You may use different flavors such as lemon lime, orange, strawberry or even a combo of all of them. You can also substitute the soda for a pitcher of powdered drink mix and 2 liters of ginger ale."

***Servings**: 15 | **Prep**: 5 m | **Ready In**: 5 m*

Ingredients

- ✓ 4 cups pineapple juice
- ✓ 1/2 gallon pineapple sherbet
- ✓ 1 liter lemon-lime flavored carbonated beverage

Directions

- ✓ Scoop all of sherbet into a large punch bowl. Add pineapple juice and soda on top of the sherbet. When adding soda the punch will foam, so make sure to stir constantly so the foam can go down. Serve immediately.

Nutritional Information

- ✓ Calories: 188 kcal 9%
- ✓ Fat: 0.1 g < 1%
- ✓ Carbs: 47g 15%
- ✓ Protein: 0.2 g < 1%
- ✓ Cholesterol: 0 mg 0%
- ✓ Sodium: 8 mg < 1%

Slime Punch

"Halloween is supposed to be horrific and gross, but this punch is spooky and sweet."

***Servings**: 16 | **Prep**: 10 m | **Ready In**: 10 m*

Ingredients

- ✓ 1 medium pumpkin (optional)
- ✓ 1/2 gallon lime sherbet
- ✓ 1 (2 liter) bottle lemon-lime soda (such as Sprite®)

Directions

- ✓ Cut the top off of the pumpkin and thoroughly scrape out the seeds and pulp. Scoop the lime sherbet into the pumpkin shell, and pour the lemon-lime soda over top.

Nutritional Information

- ✓ Calories: 212 kcal 11%
- ✓ Fat: 2.1 g 3%
- ✓ Carbs: 49.6g 16%
- ✓ Protein: 2.1 g 4%
- ✓ Cholesterol: 6 mg 2%
- ✓ Sodium: 60 mg 2%

Snow Punch

"A tart but sweet creamy punch. I often create the mixture in step 1 and save it in the refrigerator until guests arrive."

***Servings:** 12 | **Prep:** 10 m | **Ready In:** m*

Ingredients

- ✓ 6 bananas
- ✓ 2 cups half-and-half cream
- ✓ 1 cup lemon juice
- ✓ 1 cup white sugar
- ✓ 2 liters lemon-lime flavored carbonated beverage
- ✓ 1 pint lemon sherbet

Directions

1. In a blender combine bananas, half-and-half, lemon juice and sugar. Bend until smooth.

2. Pour the banana mixture into a large punch bowl. Gently stir in the carbonated beverage. Scoop out sherbet and float on top. Serve immediately.

Nutritional Information

✓ Calories: 278 kcal 14%

✓ Fat: 4.8 g 7%

✓ Carbs: 60.5g 20%

✓ Protein: 1.9 g 4%

✓ Cholesterol: 15 mg 5%

✓ Sodium: 36 mg 1%

Southern Coffee Punch

"Smooth and delicious. This is a coffee lover's dream come true."
***Servings**: 20 | **Prep**: 10 m | **Ready In**: 40 m*

Ingredients

✓ 2 cups boiling water

✓ 1 cup white sugar

✓ 1 (2 ounce) jar instant coffee granules (such as Nescafe®)

✓ 1 gallon 2% milk

✓ 1/2 gallon vanilla ice cream

✓ 1/2 gallon chocolate ice cream

Directions

1. Stir boiling water, sugar, and instant coffee together in a bowl until dissolved; cool in refrigerator, 30 minutes to overnight.

2. Pour coffee mixture into a punch bowl; add milk, vanilla ice cream, and chocolate ice cream. Stir until ice cream begins to melt.

Nutritional Information

- ✓ Calories: 363 kcal 18%
- ✓ Fat: 15.5 g 24%
- ✓ Carbs: 47.6g 15%
- ✓ Protein: 10.6 g 21%
- ✓ Cholesterol: 57 mg 19%
- ✓ Sodium: 164 mg 7%

Spicy Lemon Ginger Switchel

"This haymaker's punch is an old-timey favorite that's basically just a refreshing, palate-cleansing, vinegary, and thirst-quenching sipping drink. Pour over ice and enjoy!"

***Servings**: 1 | **Prep**: 10 m | **Ready In**: 10 m*

Ingredients

- ✓ 1 cup water
- ✓ 2 tablespoons unfiltered apple cider vinegar
- ✓ 1 tablespoon fresh lemon juice
- ✓ 4 teaspoons honey
- ✓ 1 teaspoon grated fresh ginger
- ✓ 1 pinch ground cayenne pepper

Directions

- ✓ Place water, apple cider vinegar, lemon juice, honey, fresh ginger, and cayenne pepper in a glass jar. Stir or shake well to combine.

Nutritional Information

- ✓ Calories: 103 kcal 5%
- ✓ Fat: 0 g < 1%
- ✓ Carbs: 26.6g 9%
- ✓ Protein: 0.2 g < 1%
- ✓ Cholesterol: 0 mg 0%

✓ Sodium: 10 mg < 1%

Strawberry Champagne Punch

"A simple carbonated punch with champagne, ginger ale and frozen strawberries."
*Servings: 14 | **Prep**: 5 m | **Ready In**: 5 m*

Ingredients
✓ 1 (750 milliliter) bottle champagne
✓ 1 (2 liter) bottle ginger ale, chilled
✓ 2 (10 ounce) packages frozen strawberries, partially thawed

Directions
✓ In a large punch bowl, combine champagne, ginger ale and strawberries. Gently stir and serve.

Nutritional Information
✓ Calories: 108 kcal 5%
✓ Fat: 0 g < 1%
✓ Carbs: 17.2g 6%
✓ Protein: 0.2 g < 1%
✓ Cholesterol: 0 mg 0%
✓ Sodium: 21 mg < 1%

Sugar-Free Mojito Punch

"My daughter, who has type I diabetes, came up with this sugar-free version for our Mexican-themed nights."
*Servings: 8 | **Prep**: 5 m | **Ready In**: 5 m*

Ingredients

- ✓ 1/2 cup lime juice
- ✓ 1/2 cup fresh mint leaves
- ✓ 1/4 cup granular sucralose sweetener (such as Splenda®)
- ✓ 4 1/4 cups diet lemon-lime soda
- ✓ 4 cups crushed ice

Directions

1. Stir lime juice, mint leaves, and sweetener together in a pitcher; gently crush and bruise mint leaves with a wooden spoon.
2. Pour diet lemon-lime soda into juice mixture and stir until sweetener has dissolved.
3. Mix in crushed ice to serve.

Nutritional Information

- ✓ Calories: 9 kcal < 1%
- ✓ Fat: 0 g < 1%
- ✓ Carbs: 3.7g 1%
- ✓ Protein: 0.1 g < 1%
- ✓ Cholesterol: 0 mg 0%
- ✓ Sodium: 14 mg < 1%

Tropical Orange-Guava Punch

"A light citrus punch with a tropical twist. It's very nice for weddings and receptions in the warm months, as well as for tropical-themed parties and cookouts."

Servings: 20 | **Prep**: 10 m | **Ready In**: 25 m

Ingredients

- ✓ 1 gallon orange sherbet
- ✓ 2 cups no-pulp orange juice

- ✓ 1 (12 fluid ounce) can or bottle guava nectar
- ✓ 6 liters lemon-lime soda

Directions

- ✓ Scoop sherbet into a large punch bowl. Add orange juice and guava nectar. Allow sherbet to soften for about 15 minutes, then stir to blend. Stir in lemon-lime soda just before serving.

Nutritional Information

- ✓ Calories: 136 kcal 7%
- ✓ Fat: 0.1 g < 1%
- ✓ Carbs: 35g 11%
- ✓ Protein: 0.2 g < 1%
- ✓ Cholesterol: 0 mg 0%
- ✓ Sodium: 32 mg 1%

Vanilla Punch

"Clear punch that is easy to make ahead of time, easy to serve, and wonderful tasting. Also very inexpensive to make for a large group."
Servings: *36* | **Prep:** *5 m* | **Ready In:** *5 m*

Ingredients

- ✓ 5 cups white sugar
- ✓ 2 cups water
- ✓ 2 tablespoons clear imitation vanilla extract
- ✓ 2 tablespoons almond extract

Directions

1. In a saucepan over medium heat, combine sugar and water. Cook, stirring frequently, until sugar is dissolved. Stir in vanilla and almond extract. Cool, and refrigerate.
2. To serve: In a punch bowl with ice, mix 1 cup syrup with 2 liters ginger ale or lemon-lime soda.

Note

✓ Syrup can be refrigerated for several months. If you store it in a bottle or jug, it will be easier to measure.

Nutritional Information

✓ Calories: 110 kcal 5%

✓ Fat: 0 g < 1%

✓ Carbs: 27.9g 9%

✓ Protein: 0 g < 1%

✓ Cholesterol: 0 mg 0%

✓ Sodium: < 1 mg < 1%

Warm and Spicy Autumn Punch

"The aroma of this punch tells you that fall is in the air. Make a batch, and your home will have a fragrance that will alert anyone's sense of smell."

Servings: 16 | **Prep:** 20 m | **Ready In:** 1h

Ingredients

✓ 2 oranges

✓ 8 whole cloves

✓ 6 cups apple juice

✓ 1 cinnamon stick

✓ 1/4 teaspoon ground nutmeg

✓ 1/4 cup honey

✓ 3 tablespoons lemon juice

✓ 2 1/4 cups pineapple juice

Directions

1. Preheat oven to 350 degrees F (175 degrees C). Stud the whole oranges with cloves, and bake for 30 minutes.

2. In a large saucepan, combine the apple juice and cinnamon stick. Bring to a boil, reduce heat to medium,

and simmer 5 minutes. Remove from heat, and stir in the nutmeg, honey, lemon juice, and pineapple juice.

3. Serve hot in a punch bowl with the 2 clove-studded baked oranges floating on top.

Nutritional Information

- ✓ Calories: 91 kcal 5%
- ✓ Fat: 0.2 g < 1%
- ✓ Carbs: 22.9g 7%
- ✓ Protein: 0.4 g < 1%
- ✓ Cholesterol: 0 mg 0%
- ✓ Sodium: 5 mg < 1%

Wassail Punch I

"I was given this recipe when touring a home in our community that was presented in full period costume and celebration for the Christmas holiday. In 1821 a German settler brought to the area the first tree for decorating, presented the traditional Yule Log ceremony and offered Wassail Punch."

Servings: 48 | **Prep**: 10 m | **Ready In**: 10 m

Ingredients

- ✓ 1 tablespoon whole cloves
- ✓ 6 cinnamon sticks
- ✓ 3 tablespoons chopped crystallized ginger
- ✓ 3 3/4 cups white sugar
- ✓ 2 quarts water
- ✓ 2 quarts orange juice
- ✓ 2 cups lemon juice
- ✓ 1 gallon apple cider

Directions

1. Wrap the cloves, cinnamon stick, and ginger in cheese cloth, and tie with string.
2. In a medium saucepan, combine sugar, water and spice bag. Simmer and stir until sugar dissolves. Remove from heat, and refrigerate overnight.
3. Before serving, stir in the orange juice, lemon juice, and cider. Reheat over medium low flame, and serve warm. Be careful not to boil.

Nutritional Information

- ✓ Calories: 128 kcal 6%
- ✓ Fat: 0.1 g < 1%
- ✓ Carbs: 32.5g 10%
- ✓ Protein: 0.4 g < 1%
- ✓ Cholesterol: 0 mg 0%
- ✓ Sodium: 11 mg < 1%

Wassail Punch II

"Here is a popular drink to warm you while visiting around the Christmas Tree."

Servings: 20 | Prep: 32 m | Ready In: 10 m

Ingredients

- ✓ 1 1/2 cups white sugar
- ✓ 8 whole cloves
- ✓ 3 cups water
- ✓ 3 cinnamon sticks
- ✓ 1 1/2 cups orange juice
- ✓ 1 cup lemon juice
- ✓ 1 gallon apple juice

Directions

1. In a saucepan, combine the sugar, cloves, water, and cinnamon. Bring to a boil, and continue to boil for 10 minutes. Remove from heat, cover, and allow to cool for 1 hour.

2. Stir in the orange juice, lemon juice, and apple juice. Return to the heat, and boil for 10 to 15 minutes. Remove cloves and cinnamon sticks before serving.

Nutritional Information

- ✓ Calories: 103 kcal 5%
- ✓ Fat: 0.2 g < 1%
- ✓ Carbs: 26g 8%
- ✓ Protein: 0.2 g < 1%
- ✓ Cholesterol: 0 mg 0%
- ✓ Sodium: 5 mg < 1%

Wassail Punch

"Great for holiday gatherings. Using a slow-cooker to prepare this allows the aroma to be savored for hours."
Servings: *12* | **Prep:** *5 m* | **Cook:** *8 h* | **Ready In:** *8 h 5 m*

Ingredients

- ✓ 2 quarts apple cider
- ✓ 2 cups orange juice
- ✓ 1/2 cup lemon juice
- ✓ 12 whole cloves
- ✓ 4 cinnamon sticks
- ✓ 1 pinch ground ginger
- ✓ 1 pinch ground nutmeg

Directions

✓ In a slow-cooker or a large pot over low heat, combine apple cider, orange juice and lemon juice. Season with cloves, ginger and nutmeg. Bring to a simmer. If using a slow cooker, allow to simmer all day. Serve hot.

Nutritional Information

✓ Calories: 101 kcal 5%

✓ Fat: 0.4 g < 1%

✓ Carbs: 24.9g 8%

✓ Protein: 0.5 g 1%

✓ Cholesterol: 0 mg 0%

✓ Sodium: 8 mg < 1%

Winter Punch

"An apple-orange cinnamonny hot drink."
Servings: *4 |* ***Prep:*** *2 m |* ***Cook:*** *4 m |* ***Ready In:*** *6 m*

Ingredients

✓ 2 3/4 cups apple juice

✓ 1 1/4 cups orange juice

✓ 1 tablespoon lemon juice

✓ 2 tablespoons honey

✓ 2 teaspoons ground cinnamon

Directions

✓ In a saucepan, combine apple juice and orange juice. Heat over medium heat until steaming hot, but not boiling. Remove from heat and sir in lemon juice, honey and cinnamon. Serve hot.

Nutritional Information

✓ Calories: 151 kcal 8%

✓ Fat: 0.4 g < 1%

- ✓ Carbs: 37.9g 12%
- ✓ Protein: 0.7 g 1%
- ✓ Cholesterol: 0 mg 0%
- ✓ Sodium: 6 mg < 1%

Witches' Brew

"A fun Halloween attention-getter. Great for parties. A fake hand is frozen in a disposable glove and then slipped into the punch bowl!"
Servings: *16* | **Prep:** *30 m* | **Cook:** *10 m* | **Ready In:** *7 d*

Ingredients

- ✓ 1 (10 ounce) package frozen raspberries, thawed
- ✓ 2 1/2 cups cranberry juice
- ✓ 2 envelopes unflavored gelatin
- ✓ 2 liters ginger ale
- ✓ 2 liters sparkling apple cider (non-alcoholic)
- ✓ 6 gummi snakes candy

Directions

1. To make the frozen hand: Wash and rinse the outside of a rubber glove. Turn glove inside out and set aside. In a 4 cup measuring cup, combine the thawed raspberries and cranberry juice.
2. Pour 2 cups of the raspberry mixture into a small saucepan. Sprinkle the gelatin over and let stand 2 minutes. Warm over low heat, stirring constantly, just until gelatin dissolves. Mix back into the reserved raspberry mixture in the measuring cup.
3. Pour raspberry mixture into the inverted glove. Gather up the top of the glove and tie securely with kitchen twine. Freeze until solid, or several days if possible.

4. To serve: Carefully cut glove away from frozen hand. Place frozen hand, palm side up, leaning against side of a large punch bowl. Pour in ginger ale and sparkling cider. Garnish with gummy snakes.

Editor's Note

✓ To avoid issues with people who may have allergies to latex, use a disposable glove that is latex-free. There is usually an alternative available in the cleaning department of your grocery store.

Nutritional Information

✓ Calories: 156 kcal 8%

✓ Fat: 0.1 g < 1%

✓ Carbs: 37.7g 12%

✓ Protein: 0.9 g 2%

✓ Cholesterol: 0 mg 0%

✓ Sodium: 31 mg 1%

Yummy Apple Cider Punch

"I've made this recipe twice for separate Halloween parties, and guests couldn't get enough! A delicious apple cider punch that is sure to be a hit at any autumn party."
Servings: 8 | **Prep**: 10 m | **Ready In**: 10 m

Ingredients

✓ 6 cups apple cider

✓ 1 (750 milliliter) bottle sparkling red grape juice

✓ 2 cups orange juice

✓ 2 tablespoons lemon juice, or more to taste

Directions

- ✓ Stir apple cider, sparkling grape juice or wine (see Cook's Note), orange juice, and lemon juice together and refrigerate until serving.

Cook's Note

- ✓ For an alcoholic version, 1 bottle chilled red wine or Champagne is suggested. Feel free to experiment with the flavors. For example, try orange-mango juice! Or skip the orange entirely and go for cranberry-grape juice with white white or white sparkling grape juice. The possibilities are endless! Serve chilled.

Nutritional Information

- ✓ Calories: 172 kcal 9%
- ✓ Fat: 0.1 g < 1%
- ✓ Carbs: 41.5g 13%
- ✓ Protein: 1.2 g 2%
- ✓ Cholesterol: 0 mg 0%
- ✓ Sodium: 29 mg 1%

Six: Tea Recipes

* * *

Hot Tea

* * *

Adeni Tea

"This recipe come from Aden, Yemen. Its great for a weekend brunch or breakfast. Sweet, rich, authentic, fragrant, and magical hot drink. Great for the winter."

***Servings**: 4 | **Prep**: 10 m | **Cook**: 15 m | **Ready In**: 25 m*

Ingredients

- ✓ 3 orange pekoe tea bags
- ✓ 3 cups water
- ✓ 1/4 cup white sugar
- ✓ 10 cardamom seeds, or to taste
- ✓ 1/2 teaspoon ground cinnamon
- ✓ 1/2 teaspoon ground nutmeg
- ✓ 1/2 teaspoon ground ginger
- ✓ 1 (12 fluid ounce) can evaporated milk

Directions

1. Cut tea bags open and empty into a small bowl; discard tea bags.
2. Bring water to a boil in a saucepan; add loose tea. Boil tea until water becomes dark red, 3 to 5 minutes. Stir sugar into tea.
3. Grind cardamom seeds in an electric grinder or using a mortar and pestle. Stir ground cardamom, cinnamon, nutmeg, and ginger into tea; boil until flavors are infused, about 10 minutes.

4. Stir milk into tea and bring back to a boil for about 2 minutes. Pour tea through a sieve to separate out solids. Serve hot.

Nutritional Information

- ✓ Calories: 179 kcal 9%
- ✓ Fat: 7.3 g 11%
- ✓ Carbs: 22.6g 7%
- ✓ Protein: 6.5 g 13%
- ✓ Cholesterol: 27 mg 9%
- ✓ Sodium: 106 mg 4%

Anti Allergy Tea

A tonic to help prevent or ease symptoms of hay fever and other allergies.

Ingredients

- ✓ 5 oz. nettle
- ✓ 2 oz. mullein
- ✓ 1 oz. ginger
- ✓ 1 oz. licorice
- ✓ 1 oz. peppermint
- ✓ Pinch of cayenne for warmth and flavor (optional)

Directions

1. To make blend: Combine dried herbs; mix well. Store in tightly sealed glass jar. (Dried blend will keep for up to a year.)
2. To make 1 quart tea: Pour 1 quart boiling water over 8 teaspoons blend in teapot or mason jar. Cover and steep for 15 to 20 minutes. Strain and discard herbs. Sweeten with honey if desired. Drink 3 to 4 cups daily.

Cook's Notes

- ✓ Buying Dried Herbs: High-quality dried herbs are just as potent as fresh herbs, and are generally available in bulk at natural-foods stores and in specialty herb stores.
- ✓ This recipe calls for dried herbs (not powdered dried herbs), and requires these basic tools of the trade: a kitchen scale; a fine mesh strainer; large glass jars with an airtight seal; a teapot with lid, or mason jar.

Chai Tea Mix

"Instant Chai tea mix. You can spice it up even further by adding 1 teaspoon nutmeg and allspice, and 1/4 teaspoon white pepper."
Servings: 4 | **Prep**: 30 m | **Cook**: 2 m | **Ready In**: 32 m

Ingredients

- ✓ 1 cup nonfat dry milk powder
- ✓ 1 cup powdered non-dairy creamer
- ✓ 1 cup French vanilla flavored powdered non-dairy creamer
- ✓ 2 1/2 cups white sugar
- ✓ 1 1/2 cups unsweetened instant tea
- ✓ 2 teaspoons ground ginger
- ✓ 2 teaspoons ground cinnamon
- ✓ 1 teaspoon ground cloves
- ✓ 1 teaspoon ground cardamom

Directions

1. In a large bowl, combine milk powder, non-dairy creamer, vanilla flavored creamer, sugar and instant tea. Stir in ginger, cinnamon, cloves and cardamom. In a blender or food processor, blend 1 cup at a time, until mixture is the consistency of fine powder.

2. To serve: Stir 2 heaping tablespoons Chai tea mixture into a mug of hot water.

Cook's Note

✓ You may choose to omit the French vanilla creamer, and use 2 teaspoons vanilla extract instead. To do so, mix the vanilla into the sugar, let it dry, then break the sugar into small lumps. Follow the same procedure as above.

Nutritional Information

✓ Calories: 100 kcal 5%
✓ Fat: 1.9 g 3%
✓ Carbs: 19.5g 6%
✓ Protein: 1.8 g 4%
✓ Cholesterol: < 1 mg < 1%
✓ Sodium: 28 mg 1%

Chandra Chai Moon Tea

"This recipe is the culmination of much experimentation in my kitchen. I have omitted black tea, as I am not fond of caffeine. The resulting tea follows in the tradition sprung up on the west coast, particularly the SF bay area, where a fondness for strong spices seems to be most favored, savored and brewed. Add enough soy milk or cows milk to suit your taste."

Servings: 1 | Prep: 15 m | Cook: 2 h | Ready In: 2 h 15 m

Ingredients

✓ 5 cups water
✓ 1 teaspoon whole cloves
✓ 1/2 teaspoon fennel seeds
✓ 1/2 teaspoon licorice root
✓ 1/2 teaspoon whole allspice berries
✓ 1 vanilla bean

- ✓ 3 tablespoons honey
- ✓ 2% milk

Directions

- ✓ In a saucepan, combine water, cloves, fennel seeds, licorice root, allspice berries and vanilla bean. Cover snugly and simmer over medium-low heat for 40 to 50 minutes. Filter into a suitable container and stir in honey. Stir in milk to taste.

Nutritional Information

- ✓ Calories: 77 kcal 4%
- ✓ Fat: 1 g 2%
- ✓ Carbs: 16.1 g 5%
- ✓ Protein: 1.7 g 3%
- ✓ Cholesterol: 4 mg 1%
- ✓ Sodium: 22 mg < 1%

Citrus-Honey Green Tea

"Hubby and I try to drink green tea on a daily basis. I came up with this recipe to make it more interesting. You can use freshly squeezed orange juice instead of grapefruit juice."

Servings: 1 | Prep: 10 m | Ready In: 10 m

Ingredients

- ✓ 1 (2 inch) piece lemon zest, cut into thin slivers
- ✓ 2 teaspoons boiling water
- ✓ 2 teaspoons green tea powder
- ✓ 3/4 cup hot water
- ✓ 1/2 cup freshly squeezed grapefruit juice
- ✓ 3 tablespoons freshly squeezed lemon juice
- ✓ 1 teaspoon honey

Directions

- ✓ Put lemon zest into a large cup or mug. Cover with 2 teaspoons boiling water and let steep for about 3 minutes. Stir in the green tea powder and hot water. Add the grapefruit juice, lemon juice and honey. Mix well and serve.

Nutritional Information

- ✓ Calories: 89 kcal 4%
- ✓ Fat: 0.2 g < 1%
- ✓ Carbs: 22.5g 7%
- ✓ Protein: 1.4 g 3%
- ✓ Cholesterol: 0 mg 0%
- ✓ Sodium: 9 mg < 1%

Cocoa Tea Mix Recipe

"Not everyone will be a fan of this earthy, sweet drink. Depends what tea you use really. I use Earl Grey Black Tea, but you can use any tea you love. Try out this unique drink."
Servings: 1 | **Prep**: 10 m | **Ready In**: 10 m

Ingredients

- ✓ 1 1/2 cups boiling water
- ✓ 1 Earl Grey tea bag
- ✓ 3 tablespoons milk
- ✓ 1 1/2 tablespoons hot cocoa mix
- ✓ 2 teaspoons white sugar

Directions

- ✓ Pour boiling water into a mug and steep tea bag, about 2 minutes. Remove tea bag; add milk, hot cocoa mix, and sugar. Stir until well-blended, about 20 seconds.

Cook's Note

- ✓ Use 2 tea bags if you prefer stronger tea.

Nutritional Information

- ✓ Calories: 103 kcal 5%
- ✓ Fat: 1.4 g 2%
- ✓ Carbs: 20.5g 7%
- ✓ Protein: 2.3 g 5%
- ✓ Cholesterol: 4 mg 1%
- ✓ Sodium: 90 mg 4%

Coffeebar Chai

"A delicious Chai tea that is easy to make at home. Serve hot or over ice."
Servings: 4 | **Prep**: 5 m | **Cook**: 10 m | **Ready In**: 15 m

Ingredients

- ✓ 2 cups water
- ✓ 4 black tea bags
- ✓ 1/4 cup honey
- ✓ 1/2 teaspoon vanilla extract
- ✓ 1 cinnamon stick
- ✓ 5 whole cloves
- ✓ 1/4 teaspoon ground cardamom
- ✓ 1/4 teaspoon ground ginger
- ✓ 1 pinch ground nutmeg
- ✓ 2 cups milk

Directions

- ✓ In a saucepan, bring water to a boil. Add tea, honey and vanilla. Season with cinnamon, cloves, cardamom, ginger and nutmeg. Simmer for 5 minutes. Pour in milk, and bring to a boil. Remove from heat, and strain through a fine sieve.

Nutritional Information

- ✓ Calories: 135 kcal 7%
- ✓ Fat: 2.6 g 4%
- ✓ Carbs: 24.9g 8%
- ✓ Protein: 4.2 g 8%
- ✓ Cholesterol: 10 mg 3%
- ✓ Sodium: 58 mg 2%

Common Cold Tea

Try this soothing herbal blend for a cold that rests in the lungs with a fever and dry, irritating cough.

Ingredients

- ✓ 2 1/2 oz. peppermint
- ✓ 2 1/2 oz. elder flowers
- ✓ 2 1/2 oz. yarrow
- ✓ 1 oz. mullein
- ✓ 1 oz. licorice
- ✓ 1 oz. echinacea
- ✓ 1/2 oz. ginger

Directions

1. To make blend: Combine peppermint, elder, yarrow, and mullein in glass jar. Combine licorice, echinacea, and ginger in separate jar. (Store blends in tightly sealed glass jars. Dried blends will keep for up to a year.)
2. To make 1 quart tea: Add 4 teaspoons licorice mixture to 4 to 5 cups cold water; bring to a boil and let simmer for 15 to 20 minutes, covered. Turn off heat and add 4 teaspoons of peppermint mixture; cover and steep for 15 to 20 minutes. Strain and discard herbs. Sweeten with honey if desired. Drink 1/4 cup every half-hour.

Cook's Notes

✓ Buying Dried Herbs: High-quality dried herbs are just as potent as fresh herbs, and are generally available in bulk at natural-foods stores and in specialty herb stores.

✓ This recipe calls for dried herbs (not powdered dried herbs), and requires these basic tools of the trade: a kitchen scale; a fine mesh strainer; large glass jars with an airtight seal; a teapot with lid, or mason jar.

Emerald-Drop Snow Tea

"This recipe was inspired by one of my favorite movies, Narnia: The Lion, the Witch, and the Wardrobe."
Servings: 2 | **Prep**: 10 m | **Cook**: 5 m | **Ready In**: 15 m

Ingredients

✓ 3 cups hot water
✓ 2 tablespoons Italian red wine, or more to taste
✓ 2 tablespoons white sugar
✓ 3/4 teaspoon ground cinnamon
✓ 1/4 teaspoon ground nutmeg
✓ 1/4 teaspoon ground ginger
✓ 4 fresh spearmint leaves
✓ 1 leaf fresh mint leaf
✓ 1/2 apple, cubed

Directions

✓ Combine water, red wine, sugar, cinnamon, nutmeg, ginger, spearmint leaves, and mint leaf in a saucepan; bring to a boil. Reduce heat to low and add apple to mixture. Simmer tea until apple breaks easily with a fork, about 5 minutes. Remove apple using a slotted spoon or strainer and pour tea into a mug.

Nutritional Information
- ✓ Calories: 86 kcal 4%
- ✓ Fat: 0.2 g < 1%
- ✓ Carbs: 19g 6%
- ✓ Protein: 0.3 g < 1%
- ✓ Cholesterol: 0 mg 0%
- ✓ Sodium: 13 mg < 1%

Fuss Free Hot Cranberry Tea

"I have looked for recipes for hot cranberry tea that are simple and don't involve a lot of time. This is it! My mother is a cook who adds until it tastes good. This is what she came up with. Increase or decrease quantities to suit your own taste."

Servings: 26 | **Prep**: 5 m | **Cook**: 10 m | **Ready In**: 15 m

Ingredients
- ✓ 1/2 gallon orange juice
- ✓ 1 (64 fluid ounce) bottle cranberry-raspberry juice 1 (16 ounce) can pineapple juice
- ✓ 2 (2.25 ounce) packages small red cinnamon candies
- ✓ 1/2 gallon water
- ✓ 8 tea bags

Directions
1. Combine the orange juice, cranberry-raspberry juice, pineapple juice, and cinnamon candies in a large stockpot; cook over high heat until the candies dissolve.
2. Combine the water and tea bags in a separate pot and bring to a boil; reduce heat and simmer 5 to 10 minutes; pour into juice mixture. Serve hot.

Nutritional Information
- ✓ Calories: 100 kcal 5%

- ✓ Fat: 0.2 g < 1%
- ✓ Carbs: 24.3g 8%
- ✓ Protein: 0.6 g 1%
- ✓ Cholesterol: 0 mg 0%
- ✓ Sodium: 7 mg < 1%

Genmai-cha

"Once upon a time, tea was expensive. This became a way of stretching money and still tastes great."

Servings: 4 | **Prep**: 1 m | **Cook**: 10 m | **Ready In**: 11 m

Ingredients

- ✓ 2 tablespoons brown rice
- ✓ 4 cups water
- ✓ 4 teaspoons green tea leaves

Directions

- ✓ Put the rice in a small skillet and toast over medium-low heat until it turns dark in spots. Move to a small saucepan. Pour in the water and bring to a boil. Immediately reduce heat to low; cover and simmer 1 minute. Remove from heat and allow to steep 3 minutes more. Add the tea and let it steep another 3 minutes. Strain and discard the rice and tea leaves from the liquid. Serve the tea hot.

Nutritional Information

- ✓ Calories: 24 kcal 1%
- ✓ Fat: 0.2 g < 1%
- ✓ Carbs: 4.9g 2%
- ✓ Protein: 0.7 g 1%
- ✓ Cholesterol: 0 mg 0%
- ✓ Sodium: 8 mg < 1%

Ginger-Turmeric Herbal Tea

"If you are having trouble including these anti-inflammatory spices in your diet, here is an alternative to supplements. Actually quite tasty! I believe this tea is popular in Okinawa, Japan. Just remember turmeric stains. I make mine in an old mason jar, wrapped in an old tea towel! Turmeric is used for medicinal purposes in India."

***Servings**: 1 | **Prep**: 5 m | **Cook**: 15 m | **Ready In**: 20 m*

Ingredients

- ✓ 2 cups water
- ✓ 1/2 teaspoon ground turmeric
- ✓ 1/2 teaspoon chopped fresh ginger
- ✓ 1/2 teaspoon ground cinnamon (optional)
- ✓ 1 tablespoon honey
- ✓ 1 lemon wedge

Directions

- ✓ Bring water to a boil in a small saucepan; add turmeric, ginger, and cinnamon. Reduce heat to medium-low and simmer for 10 minutes. Strain tea into a large glass; add honey and lemon wedge.

Cook's Note

- ✓ Maple syrup can be substituted for the honey, if desired.

Nutritional Information

- ✓ Calories: 100 kcal 5%
- ✓ Fat: 2.6 g 4%
- ✓ Carbs: 14.6g 5%
- ✓ Protein: 5 g 10%
- ✓ Cholesterol: 10 mg 3%
- ✓ Sodium: 55 mg 2%

'Good for What Ails Ya' Tomato Tea

"This is a recipe my husband found and adapted. It is supposed to be good for clearing your sinuses, but we love it as a warm winter treat. Use any hot sauce you like; we have found the fruitier ones taste best. This also makes a great Bloody Mary mix. Serve in mugs, with a stick of celery."

Servings: *2* | ***Prep***: *10 m* | ***Cook***: *5 m* | ***Ready In***: *15 m*

Ingredients

- ✓ 3 cups tomato juice
- ✓ 1 tablespoon minced garlic
- ✓ 1 tablespoon lemon juice
- ✓ 1 tablespoon hot sauce
- ✓ 1/2 teaspoon celery salt
- ✓ 1 pinch ground black pepper

Directions

1. Blend tomato juice, garlic, lemon juice, hot sauce, celery salt, and black pepper together in a blender on low until smooth. Pour tomato juice mixture into a saucepan.
2. Heat tomato juice mixture in the saucepan over medium heat until just simmering, about 5 minutes.

Nutritional Information

- ✓ Calories: 73 kcal 4%
- ✓ Fat: 0.3 g < 1%
- ✓ Carbs: 18g 6%
- ✓ Protein: 3.2 g 6%
- ✓ Cholesterol: 0 mg 0%
- ✓ Sodium: 1537 mg 61%

Green Tea Lemonade

Who doesn't love green tea and all of its amazing health benefits? Indulge in a glass of this green tea lemonade and feel the antioxidants surge through your body.

Ingredients

- ✓ 4 bags organic green tea
- ✓ 10 cups filtered water
- ✓ ¼ teaspoon concentrated stevia powder *see note
- ✓ ½ cup + 1 tablespoon fresh lemon juice

Directions

1. Place water in a large saucepan, cover, and heat on high heat until boiling. Remove from heat and drop in teabags. Allow to steep for 10-15 minutes.
2. Remove tea bags and stir in honey, mixing until dissolved. Allow pot to sit for a couple of hours to cool before pouring into a large glass jug, mixing in lemon juice, and storing in the fridge until use.

Green Tea with Lemon and Pomegranate

Pomegranate seeds, rich in plant compounds, enhance the already potent antioxidant activity in a hot cup of green tea with lemon and honey.

Servings: 2

Ingredients

- ✓ 2 teaspoons green tea (or 2 tea bags)
- ✓ 2 cups boiling water
- ✓ 2 thin slices smashed ginger
- ✓ 1 to 2 lemon wedges
- ✓ 1/4 cup lightly crushed pomegranate seeds
- ✓ 2 tablespoons honey or sugar to taste

Directions

    ✓ Cover green tea with boiling water, ginger, lemon wedges, pomegranate seeds, and honey. Let tea steep for 3 to 5 minutes and remove.

Herbal Tea

"This recipe makes a nice tea on a cold day." in refrigerator and reheat as needed."

Servings*: 4 |* **Prep***: 5 m |* **Cook***: 2 m |* **Ready In***: 30 m*

Ingredients

    ✓ 1 quart water, or as needed
    ✓ 1 tablespoon honey
    ✓ 1 teaspoon ground cumin
    ✓ 1 teaspoon grated fresh ginger
    ✓ 1 teaspoon grated lime zest
    ✓ 1 teaspoon lime juice
    ✓ 3 leaves fresh mint

Directions

    ✓ Bring water to a boil in a pot; stir in honey, cumin, ginger, lime zest, lime juice, and mint. Cook and stir until flavors are infused, about 2 minutes.

Cook's Note

    ✓ Use the zest and juice of a lemon instead of a lime, if desired.

Nutritional Information

    ✓ Calories: 19 kcal < 1%
    ✓ Fat: 0.1 g < 1%
    ✓ Carbs: 4.8g 2%
    ✓ Protein: 0.1 g < 1%
    ✓ Cholesterol: 0 mg 0%

✓ Sodium: 8 mg < 1%

Hibiscus Tea Sparkler

Serving: 4 | Total Time: 25 mins

Ingredients

- ✓ 6 ounces boiling water
- ✓ 3 hibiscus tea bags
- ✓ 2 cups sparkling water
- ✓ 2 drops liquid Stevia or preferred sweetener to taste (optional)
- ✓ 1/2 cup raspberries, blackberries, and/or blueberries
- ✓ Juice of 1/2 lemon (optional)
- ✓ Pineapple for garnish (optional)
- ✓ Ice cubes

Directions

- ✓ Pour boiling water over tea bags and brew 5 minutes. Chill tea in the freezer or refrigerator (careful not to crack the glass!) until room temperature or colder. Remove tea bags and pour into a pitcher or large jar. Add sparkling water, berries, lemon, sweetener if desired, and ice cubes. For pineapple stars, slice pineapple about 1/4-inch thick and punch stars out with a cookie cutter.

Honey-Lemon Ginger Tea

"I visited a coffee shop in Hartford on a cold winter day and ordered their honey lemon ginger tea. It was tart, sweet, full of flavor, and warmed me from head to toe. The proprietor was nice enough to give me a rough description of her recipe. After a few tries at home, I came up with this

close version."
*Servings: 6 | **Prep**: 5 m | **Cook**: 20 m | **Ready In**: 30 m*

Ingredients

- ✓ 4 cups water
- ✓ 3/4 cup brown sugar
- ✓ 1/4 cup grated ginger root
- ✓ 3 tea bags
- ✓ 2 lemons, juiced
- ✓ 3 tablespoons honey

Directions

1. Stir water, brown sugar, and grated ginger root together in a saucepan; bring to a boil, reduce heat to medium-low, and cook at a simmer for 20 minutes.
2. Remove saucepan from heat and add tea bags; steep tea to desired strength, 3 to 5 minutes. Remove and discard tea bags.
3. Stir lemon juice and honey into the tea; strain into a pitcher.

Nutritional Information

- ✓ Calories: 104 kcal 5%
- ✓ Fat: 0 g < 1%
- ✓ Carbs: 27.1g 9%
- ✓ Protein: 0.1 g < 1%
- ✓ Cholesterol: 0 mg 0%
- ✓ Sodium: 11 mg < 1%

Hot Chai Latte

"A delicious, warm, old-fashioned style Chai Tea. With yummy spices, and authentic flavors, it's bound to be a hit with the whole family!"
*Servings: 2 | **Prep**: 5 m | **Cook**: 10 m | **Ready In**: 15 m*

Ingredients

- ✓ 1 cup milk
- ✓ 1 cup water
- ✓ 1 large strip of orange peel
- ✓ 3 whole cloves
- ✓ 1 (3 inch) cinnamon stick
- ✓ 3 whole black peppercorns
- ✓ 1 pinch ground nutmeg
- ✓ 4 teaspoons white sugar
- ✓ 2 teaspoons black tea leaves

Directions

- ✓ Combine the milk and water in a saucepan over medium-high heat. Once this mixture has warmed, place the orange peel, cloves, cinnamon stick, peppercorns, nutmeg, sugar and tea leaves into the pan. Bring to a boil, then reduce heat to medium-low, and simmer until the color deepens to your liking. Strain out spices, and pour into cups.

Nutritional Information

- ✓ Calories: 111 kcal 6%
- ✓ Fat: 2.8 g 4%
- ✓ Carbs: 17.9g 6%
- ✓ Protein: 4.6 g 9%
- ✓ Cholesterol: 10 mg 3%
- ✓ Sodium: 55 mg 2%

Hot Cranberry Tea

"A sentimental favorite. My mother and I made it when I was 7 and it's been a part of our holiday tradition ever since. A fun recipe to make with the kids. A slow cooker will keep it warm while serving."

*Servings: 14 | **Cook**: 15 m | **Ready In**: 1 h 30 m*

Ingredients

- ✓ 3 1/2 quarts water
- ✓ 1 (12 ounce) package cranberries
- ✓ 2 cups white sugar
- ✓ 2 oranges, juiced
- ✓ 2 lemons, juiced
- ✓ 12 whole cloves
- ✓ 2 cinnamon sticks

Directions

- ✓ In a large pot, combine water and cranberries. Bring to a boil, reduce heat, and simmer for 30 minutes. Add sugar, orange juice, lemon juice, cloves and cinnamon sticks. Cover, and steep for 1 hour.

Nutritional Information

- ✓ Calories: 140 kcal 7%
- ✓ Fat: 0.2 g < 1%
- ✓ Carbs: 36.8g 12%
- ✓ Protein: 0.6 g 1%
- ✓ Cholesterol: 0 mg 0%
- ✓ Sodium: 10 mg < 1%

Hot Spiced Tea for the Holidays

"This is an old family favorite, handed down from my great-grandmother. The holidays officially begin with Christmas carols and my favorite hot spiced tea! Definitely a seasonal comfort beverage for me! I prefer to use fresh juices with pulp. The flavors are different. Canned pineapple in light syrup is best. Set the pineapple chunks aside for the rest of your holiday baking. Store leftovers in refrigerator and reheat as needed."

*Servings: 6 | **Prep**: 5 m | **Cook**: 10 m | **Ready In**: 30 m*

Ingredients

- ✓ 6 cups water
- ✓ 1 teaspoon whole cloves
- ✓ 1 (1 inch) piece cinnamon stick
- ✓ 6 tea bags (such as Lipton®)
- ✓ 3/4 cup orange juice
- ✓ 1/2 cup white sugar
- ✓ 1/4 cup pineapple juice
- ✓ 2 tablespoons lemon juice

Directions

1. Pour water into a pot; add cloves and cinnamon stick. Bring water to a boil; remove from heat. Add tea bags to water and set aside to steep until the tea is to your preferred strength, at least 5 minutes. Remove and discard cloves, cinnamon stick, and tea bags.

2. Stir orange juice, sugar, pineapple juice, and lemon juice together in a saucepan; bring to a boil. Cook and stir the juice mixture until the sugar dissolves completely. Pour juice mixture into the spiced tea; serve hot.

Nutritional Information

- ✓ Calories: 87 kcal 4%
- ✓ Fat: 0.1 g < 1%
- ✓ Carbs: 22g 7%
- ✓ Protein: 0.3 g < 1%
- ✓ Cholesterol: 0 mg 0%
- ✓ Sodium: 9 mg < 1%

Hot Spiced Tea

This sweet, gingery tea is a perfect way to start your morning, maybe with a pistachio raisin biscotti.

*Servings: 4 | **Prep**: 5 mins | **Total time**: 25 mins*

Ingredients

- ✓ 3 cups water
- ✓ 1 1/2-inch piece fresh ginger, unpeeled, halved lengthwise
- ✓ 4 tea bags (such as black tea)
- ✓ 1 cinnamon stick, plus 4 for garnish
- ✓ 8 whole cloves
- ✓ 1/4 teaspoon whole black peppercorns
- ✓ 2 cups low-fat milk (2 percent)
- ✓ 1/4 cup honey (or to taste)

Directions

1. In a large saucepan, bring water and fresh ginger to a boil. Reduce heat; simmer 8 minutes.
2. Add tea bags, 1 cinnamon stick, whole cloves, whole black peppercorns, and low-fat milk. Steep over medium-low heat until fragrant, about 6 minutes.
3. Strain through a sieve; discard solids. Stir in 1/4 cup honey (or to taste). Divide among mugs. Serve hot, garnished with more cinnamon sticks, if desired.

Indian Chai Hot Chocolate

"I whipped up this delicious hot chocolate in my kitchen one day when I couldn't decide on a mug of hot chocolate or chai tea latte. It tastes just like Christmas!"

*Servings: 1 | **Prep**: 2 m | **Cook**: 3 m | **Ready In**: 5 m*

Ingredients

- ✓ 1/2 cup water
- ✓ 1/2 cup milk

- ✓ 1 chai tea bag
- ✓ 1 (.55 ounce) package instant hot chocolate mix

Directions

- ✓ Stir the water and milk together in a microwave-safe mug. Cook on high in the microwave for 1 1/2 minutes. Remove, and add the chai teabag. Allow tea to steep about 2 minutes. Remove the tea bag, and stir in the hot chocolate mix.

Nutritional Information

- ✓ Calories: 126 kcal 6%
- ✓ Fat: 3 g 5%
- ✓ Carbs: 19.3g 6%
- ✓ Protein: 5.1 g 10%
- ✓ Cholesterol: 10 mg 3%
- ✓ Sodium: 131 mg 5%

Lavender Mint Tea

"This mood-boosting tea is delicious hot or iced. And fresh lavender and mint from the garden make it even more special!"
Servings: 4 | **Prep**: 5 m | **Cook**: 15 m | **Ready** In: 20 m

Ingredients

- ✓ 1/4 cup fresh lavender petals
- ✓ 1 cup fresh mint leaves
- ✓ 4 cups water

Directions

- ✓ Place lavender petals and mint leaves into a saucepan, pour water over lavender and mint, and bring to a boil. Turn heat to low and simmer tea until flavor is your desired strength, 15 to 20 minutes. Strain out mint and lavender petals and serve tea hot. If you prefer, let strained tea cool serve over ice.

Nutritional Information

- ✓ Calories: 4 kcal < 1%
- ✓ Fat: 0.1 g < 1%
- ✓ Carbs: 0.7g < 1%
- ✓ Protein: 0.3 g < 1%
- ✓ Cholesterol: 0 mg 0%
- ✓ Sodium: 9 mg < 1%

Lemon Spice Wellness Tea

"This is a classic throw-in-what-you've-got tea that will kick a cold where it hurts: in the throat. It is made with whole ingredients and no sugar - a sure sign you're on your way to wellness."

Servings: 6 | **Prep**: m | **Cook**: 10 m | **Ready In**: 10 m

Ingredients

- ✓ 6 cups water, or as desired
- ✓ 1 (4 inch) piece fresh ginger, peeled and coarsely chopped
- ✓ 1 whole star anise pod
- ✓ 6 cardamom pods, bruised
- ✓ 1 cinnamon stick
- ✓ 4 lemons
- ✓ 3 tablespoons unpasteurized honey, or more to taste

Directions

1. Bring water to a boil in a saucepan; add ginger, star anise, cardamom pods, and cinnamon stick. Zest lemons over the saucepan. Slice lemons in half and squeeze juice into the water. Reduce heat to medium-low and simmer until desired flavor is reached, 5 to 15 minutes.

2. Stir honey into tea and strain tea through a fine-mesh strainer as you ladle into mugs. Add contents in strainer back into saucepan.

Cook's Note

✓ Keep adding water and honey all day if you're committed to kicking a cold! Get better soon!

Nutritional Information

✓ Calories: 55 kcal 3%

✓ Fat: 0.3 g < 1%

✓ Carbs: 18.4g 6%

✓ Protein: 1.1 g 2%

✓ Cholesterol: 0 mg 0%

✓ Sodium: 10 mg < 1%

Lemon Verbena Mint Detox Tea

"This is a simple detox tea. Lemon verbena is delicious! I came across it while I was picking up my summer herb plants last spring. I had never heard of it before but learned it is good for cooking and tea. Little did I know this little herb has some amazing detox and medicinal benefits. I love lemon but hate what the acid does to my teeth. With lemon verbena you get the flavor of lemon without the acid."

***Servings:** 1 | **Prep:** 5 m | **Cook:** 3 m | **Ready In:** 8 m*

Ingredients

✓ 1 cup boiling water

✓ 1 sprig fresh lemon verbena (about 10 leaves)

✓ 1 sprig fresh mint (about 15 leaves)

✓ 1 teaspoon honey, or to taste (optional)

Directions

- ✓ Pour boiling water over verbena and mint sprigs; steep until desired flavor is reached, 3 to 4 minutes. Stir in honey.

Cook's Note

- ✓ I keep the leaves on the stem so that I can quickly pull them out right before enjoying; no straining necessary.

Nutritional Information

- ✓ Calories: 25 kcal 1%
- ✓ Fat: 0 g < 1%
- ✓ Carbs: 6.4g 2%
- ✓ Protein: 0.2 g < 1%
- ✓ Cholesterol: 0 mg 0%
- ✓ Sodium: 8 mg < 1%

Masala Chai

"This chai tea is hot, spicy, and has a hint of the exotic...gotta love it!"
***Servings:** 1 | **Prep:** 5 m | **Cook:** 10 m | **Ready In:** 10 m*

Ingredients

- ✓ 1 cup water
- ✓ 1 1/2 teaspoons sugar
- ✓ 1 whole cardamom pod
- ✓ 1 whole clove
- ✓ 2 black peppercorns
- ✓ 3 teaspoons black tea leaves
- ✓ 1/2 cup warm milk

Directions

- ✓ Combine the water and sugar in a small saucepan, and bring to a boil. Add the cardamom pod, clove, peppercorns and tea leaves. Remove from heat, and let the mixture steep for 2 to 3 minutes. Strain into a cup, and fill cup the rest of the way with milk. Sit back, relax, and enjoy!

Nutritional Information

- ✓ Calories: 100 kcal 5%
- ✓ Fat: 2.6 g 4%
- ✓ Carbs: 14.6g 5%
- ✓ Protein: 5 g 10%
- ✓ Cholesterol: 10 mg 3%
- ✓ Sodium: 55 mg 2%

Masala Spicy Tea

"Deliciously fragrant, sweet and tasty Eastern tea."
Servings: 3 | **Prep**: 15 m | **Cook**: 15 m | **Ready In**: 15 m

Ingredients

- ✓ 2 cups water
- ✓ 2 tea bags
- ✓ 1 whole black peppercorn
- ✓ 2 cinnamon sticks
- ✓ 2 whole cardamom pods
- ✓ 2 whole cloves
- ✓ 1/2 cup sweetened condensed milk

Directions

1. Bring the water to a boil in a saucepan over high heat. Reduce the heat to medium, and stir in the tea bags, peppercorn, cinnamon sticks, cardamom pods, and cloves. Let boil for 1 minute.
2. Pour in the condensed milk, and bring back to a boil. Remove from the heat, strain into cups, and serve.

Nutritional Information

- ✓ Calories: 174 kcal 9%
- ✓ Fat: 4.5 g 7%
- ✓ Carbs: 30.5g 10%
- ✓ Protein: 4.3 g 9%
- ✓ Cholesterol: 17 mg 6%
- ✓ Sodium: 72 mg 3%

Perfect Vanilla Tea

"This is a delicious blend of plain tea, wonderful vanilla, and spices to create the perfect mug for late night, morning, or really any time of day at all!"

Servings: 1 | **Prep**: 5 m | **Ready In**: 5 m

Ingredients

- ✓ 1 cup boiling water
- ✓ 1 orange pekoe tea bag
- ✓ 2 tablespoons milk
- ✓ 1 teaspoon white sugar (optional)
- ✓ 1/2 teaspoon vanilla extract
- ✓ 1/2 teaspoon ground cinnamon

Directions

1. Pour boiling water into a mug. Steep tea bag in water for 3 minutes; remove and discard.
2. Stir milk, sugar, vanilla extract, and cinnamon into the tea.

Nutritional Information

- ✓ Calories: 40 kcal 2%
- ✓ Fat: 0.6 g < 1%
- ✓ Carbs: 6.8g 2%
- ✓ Protein: 1.1 g 2%

✓ Cholesterol: 2 mg < 1%
✓ Sodium: 20 mg < 1%

Quick Warm Grapefruit Tea

Sweet and tart, this tea is energizing and delicious.
***Servings**: 4 | **Prep**: 10 mins | **Total time**: 10 mins*

Ingredients

✓ 2 cups fresh Ruby Red grapefruit juice (squeezed from 2 grapefruits)
✓ 2 to 4 tablespoons honey
✓ 1 cinnamon stick
✓ 1/2 teaspoon whole allspice berries

Directions

✓ In a medium pot, combine juice, honey, cinnamon, allspice, and 1/2 cup water. Bring to a boil over high heat; strain and discard solids. Serve with a grapefruit segment or strip of zest.

Railroad-Style Chai

"Indian Railroad-style Chai: this is the real stuff served out of trays and passed through the windows at railroad stops all over India. If you can find mamri tea pearls from India, use 1/4 cup of that in place of the tea bags."
***Servings**: 4 | **Prep**: 5 m | **Cook**: 5 m | **Ready In**: 10 m*

Ingredients

✓ 2 cups water
✓ 1 tablespoon fennel seed
✓ 4 whole cloves, or more to taste

- ✓ 1 1/2 teaspoons cardamom seeds
- ✓ 2 cups whole milk
- ✓ 4 black tea bags, or more to taste
- ✓ 1 tablespoon white sugar, or to taste

Directions

1. Bring water to a boil in a saucepan; add fennel, cloves, and cardamom. Continue boiling water for 3 minutes.
2. Stir milk into the water and return mixture to a low boil; add tea bags, reduce heat to low, and boil until the tea has a strong, but not bitter flavor, 2 to 3 minutes.
3. Strain tea into 4 tea mugs; sweeten with sugar to individual tastes.

Cook's Note

- ✓ It's important to use a cheap granulated tea. For years I tried to make this using the best Darjeeling and Asaam teas that I could find and it never came out right. The cheap granulated tea (basically what we put in tea bags) is the key. It takes a strong-flavored tea to stand up to the flavor imparted by the spices.

Nutritional Information

- ✓ Calories: 96 kcal 5%
- ✓ Fat: 4.3 g 7%
- ✓ Carbs: 10.5g 3%
- ✓ Protein: 4.3 g 9%
- ✓ Cholesterol: 12 mg 4%
- ✓ Sodium: 56 mg 2%

Russian Tea I

"This is a fragrant hot beverage tailor-made for the holidays. The scent of cloves and cinnamon will perfume your home."

Servings: *8 |* ***Prep****: 5 m |* ***Ready In****: 5 m*

Ingredients

- ✓ 1/2 teaspoon ground cinnamon
- ✓ 1/2 teaspoon ground ginger
- ✓ 1/2 teaspoon ground allspice
- ✓ 1/3 teaspoon ground cloves
- ✓ 1 cup white sugar
- ✓ 2 (6 ounce) cans frozen orange juice concentrate
- ✓ 1 1/2 lemons, juiced
- ✓ 8 cups water
- ✓ 1 tablespoon orange zest

Directions

1. In a large saucepan, bring 2 cups of water to a boil. Remove from heat, then stir in ground cinnamon, ground ginger, allspice, and ground cloves. Allow mixture to steep for 10 minutes.
2. Prepare frozen orange juice concentrate according to the Directions on the can.
3. Dissolve 1 cup of sugar in 1 cup of water, and stir into spice mixture. Mix in orange juice, lemon juice, and 5 cups water. Heat through. Serve with a garnish of orange zest.

Nutritional Information

- ✓ Calories: 188 kcal 9%
- ✓ Fat: 0.2 g < 1%
- ✓ Carbs: 48g 15%
- ✓ Protein: 1.6 g 3%
- ✓ Cholesterol: 0 mg 0%
- ✓ Sodium: 3 mg < 1%

Russian Tea II

"A great drink for a cold night. You can store this tea mix in a jar and give it as a gift! "
Servings: 40 | ***Prep***: 5 m | ***Ready In***: 5 m

Ingredients

- ✓ 2 cups instant tea with lemon-flavoring dry mix
- ✓ 2 cups orange-flavored drink mix (e.g. Tang)
- ✓ 1 cup white sugar
- ✓ 1 teaspoon ground cinnamon
- ✓ 1/2 teaspoon ground cloves

Directions

- ✓ In a bowl, mix together tea, orange-flavored drink mix, sugar, cinnamon and cloves. To serve place 2 tablespoons mix in a cup and fill with 8 ounces hot water.

Nutritional Information

- ✓ Calories: 91 kcal 5%
- ✓ Fat: 0 g < 1%
- ✓ Carbs: 23.7g 8%
- ✓ Protein: 0.1 g < 1%
- ✓ Cholesterol: 0 mg 0%
- ✓ Sodium: 1 mg < 1%

Russian Tea

"I love this tangy beverage on a cold winter's morning when I want something tasty and hot, but don't want coffee! It makes a great gift from your kitchen, too! If calories are your concern, use an artificially sweetened orange drink mix, eliminate the sugar and sweeten to taste with sugar substitute."
Servings: 40 | ***Prep***: 10 m | ***Ready In***: 10 m

Ingredients

- ✓ 1 cup instant tea powder
- ✓ 2 cups orange-flavored drink mix (e.g. Tang)
- ✓ 1 (3 ounce) package powdered lemonade mix
- ✓ 2 cups white sugar
- ✓ 2 teaspoons ground cinnamon
- ✓ 1/2 teaspoon ground cloves

Directions

1. In a large bowl, combine instant tea powder, orange drink mix, lemonade powder, sugar, cinnamon and cloves. Mix thoroughly. Store in a sealed jar.
2. To use, mix 3 to 4 tablespoons of mix with 1 cup hot or cold water. Adjust to taste.

Nutritional Information

- ✓ Calories: 102 kcal 5%
- ✓ Fat: 0 g < 1%
- ✓ Carbs: 26.4g 9%
- ✓ Protein: 0 g < 1%
- ✓ Cholesterol: 0 mg 0%
- ✓ Sodium: 2 mg < 1%

Shemakes Instant Chai Tea

"I have searched for an instant chai recipe on the net, but could not find one. This is what I made up, hope you enjoy it. Please feel free to modify it or adapt it."

*Servings: 48 | **Prep**: 15 m | **Ready In**: 15 m*

Ingredients

- ✓ 1 1/2 cups instant tea powder
- ✓ 2 cups powdered non-dairy creamer

- ✓ 1/2 cup dry milk powder
- ✓ 1 cup confectioners' sugar
- ✓ 1/4 cup brown sugar
- ✓ 1 teaspoon ground ginger
- ✓ 1 teaspoon ground cinnamon
- ✓ 1 teaspoon ground cloves
- ✓ 1 teaspoon ground cardamom
- ✓ 1 teaspoon ground allspice
- ✓ 1 teaspoon vanilla powder

Directions

1. In a food processor, combine instant tea, powdered creamer, milk powder, confectioners' sugar and brown sugar. Add ginger, cinnamon, cloves, cardamom, allspice and vanilla powder. Process for 2 minutes. Store in an airtight container.
2. To serve, place 4 teaspoonfuls in a mug, and fill with hot water; stir.

Nutritional Information

- ✓ Calories: 47 kcal 2%
- ✓ Fat: 1.8 g 3%
- ✓ Carbs: 7.2g 2%
- ✓ Protein: 0.8 g 2%
- ✓ Cholesterol: 1 mg < 1%
- ✓ Sodium: 13 mg < 1%

Slow Cooker Chai

"Easy version of chai tea, using whole spices and sweetened condensed milk. To vary the flavor, try adding a bit of star anise, fennel, allspice, vanilla bean, or nutmeg. For a sweeter tea, stir in a bit of brown sugar."

Servings: 4 | **Prep**: 15 m | **Cook**: 8 h 5 m | **Ready In**: 8 h 20 m

Ingredients

- ✓ 3 1/2 quarts water
- ✓ 15 slices fresh ginger, peeled
- ✓ 15 green cardamom pods, split open and seeded
- ✓ 25 whole cloves
- ✓ 3 cinnamon sticks
- ✓ 3 whole black peppercorns
- ✓ 8 black tea bags
- ✓ 1 (14 ounce) can sweetened condensed milk

Directions

1. Pour water into the crock of a slow cooker. Stir in the ginger, cardamom pods, cloves, cinnamon sticks, and peppercorns. Turn to High; simmer for 8 hours.
2. Steep tea bags in the hot spiced water for 5 minutes. Strain tea into a clean container. Stir in sweetened condensed milk; serve hot.

Easy Cleanup

- ✓ Try using a liner in your slow cooker for easier cleanup.

Nutritional Information

- ✓ Calories: 90 kcal 4%
- ✓ Fat: 2.3 g 3%
- ✓ Carbs: 15.6g 5%
- ✓ Protein: 2.2 g 4%
- ✓ Cholesterol: 8 mg 3%
- ✓ Sodium: 42 mg 2%

Soothing Ginger Tea

Mint invigorates a calming tea, brewed from a traditional Indian blend of ginger, fennel, and cardamom.

Servings: *4*

Ingredients

- ✓ 4 1/2 teaspoons cardamom pods, crushed
- ✓ 4 1/2 teaspoons fennel seeds
- ✓ 5 cups water
- ✓ 1 piece (6 inches) fresh ginger, peeled and sliced inch thick (about 3/4 cup)
- ✓ 1 tablespoon honey
- ✓ 1/3 cup fresh mint leaves, plus sprigs for garnish

Directions

1. Toast cardamom and fennel in a saucepan over medium-high heat for 1 minute. Add water and ginger. Reduce heat, and simmer until it reaches the desired strength, 10 to 15 minutes.
2. Remove from heat, and stir in honey and mint leaves. Let stand for 5 minutes. Strain into mugs. Garnish with mint.

Spiced Tea Mix

"This is a delicious dry spiced tea mix which can be packed in jars and given as gifts. It can also be prepared sugar free by using sugar free orange flavored drink mix and sugar free iced tea mix."

Servings: *6*

Ingredients

- ✓ 1 (3 ounce) package lemon-flavored ice tea mix 2 (1.8 ounce) packages orange-flavored drink mix (e.g. Tang) 1 1/3 tablespoons ground cinnamon 2 teaspoons ground cloves

Directions

1. Combine iced tea mix, orange flavored drink mix, ground cinnamon, and ground cloves. Store in an airtight container.
2. To serve, stir 1 1/2 teaspoon mix into 1 cup hot water.

Nutritional Information

- ✓ Calories: 116 kcal 6%
- ✓ Fat: 0.2 g < 1%
- ✓ Carbs: 29.2g 9%
- ✓ Protein: 1.1 g 2%
- ✓ Cholesterol: 0 mg 0%
- ✓ Sodium: 11 mg < 1%

Stress Soother Tea

A gentle blend of herbs that can be sipped all day long to calm nerves and ease anxiety.

Ingredients

- ✓ 3 3/4 oz. chamomile
- ✓ 4 oz. lemon balm
- ✓ 1 oz. oat tops
- ✓ 1 oz. mixed hawthorn berries and leaf/flower (sold separately)
- ✓ Stevia leaf, organic rose petals, and orange peel as desired

Directions

1. To make blend: Combine dried herbs; mix well. Store in tightly sealed glass jar. (Dried blend will keep for up to a year.)
2. To make 1 quart tea: Pour 1 quart boiling water over 8 teaspoons blend in teapot or mason jar. Cover and steep

for 15 to 20 minutes; strain and discard herbs. Drink 3 to 4 cups daily.

Throat Coat Tea

"We have all had those days when we have a cold and can't kick its butt. Where our throat is achy and it hurts to swallow. This is a recipe I have developed in the last couple of days. I think I now have the perfect balance of home-remedy qualities and flavor. The honey coats your throat and helps to sooth it. The citrus actually reduces the swelling and adds a great deal of flavor. For all of you who are suffering with a sore throat, get well soon. I hope you like it."

Servings: 1 | Prep: 5 m | Ready In: 10 m

Ingredients

- ✓ Water
- ✓ 2 (1/4-inch-thick) lemon slices
- ✓ 1 tablespoon loose-leaf jasmine green tea
- ✓ 1 teaspoon honey, or to taste

Directions

1. Heat water to near boiling in a kettle.
2. Put lemon slices, tea leaves, and honey into a mug. Pour water into the mug.
3. Steep tea until the flavor is to your liking, 3 to 5 minutes.

Nutritional Information

- ✓ Calories: 36 kcal 2%
- ✓ Fat: 0.2 g < 1%
- ✓ Carbs: 10.3g 3%
- ✓ Protein: 1.1 g 2%
- ✓ Cholesterol: 0 mg 0%
- ✓ Sodium: 10 mg < 1%

Thyme Tea

Teatime? Try this thyme tea (actually a tisane). The herb gets steeped with coriander and fennel seeds -- a nice break from the usual herbal tea assortments.

Servings: *4* | **Prep Time**: *10 mins*| **Total Time**: *20 mins*

Ingredients
- ✓ 3 cups water
- ✓ 8 to 10 thin, tender thyme sprigs
- ✓ 1/2 teaspoon whole coriander seeds, lightly crushed
- ✓ 1/2 teaspoon whole fennel seeds, lightly crushed

Directions
- ✓ Bring water to a boil. Steep thyme and the coriander and fennel seeds for 10 minutes. Strain through a fine sieve. Serve warm or chilled.

Ultimate Cold Relief Home Remedy Tea

"If you feel it coming on drink lots of this. It can't hurt, and seems to have some effect clearing nasal passages. You may hate it at first, but by the end of the first cup you may want to make more. Breath the steam in deeply. Drink it as much or as often as possible while fighting off your cold. You can substitute balsamic vinegar for the apple cider vinegar"

Servings: *1* | **Prep**: *10 m* | **Ready In**: *10 m*

Ingredients
- ✓ 8 ounces water, or as needed
- ✓ 1 tablespoon apple cider vinegar
- ✓ 1 tablespoon honey
- ✓ 1 cinnamon stick
- ✓ 1 clove garlic, peeled and smashed

Directions

- ✓ Combine water, vinegar, honey, cinnamon stick, and garlic in a small saucepan. Heat to 100 degrees F (38 degrees C); remove from heat and pour into a mug.

Nutritional Information

- ✓ Calories: 79 kcal 4%
- ✓ Fat: 0.1 g < 1%
- ✓ Carbs: 21g 7%
- ✓ Protein: 0.4 g < 1%
- ✓ Cholesterol: 0 mg 0%
- ✓ Sodium: 9 mg < 1%

Women's Balancing Tea

A regulating formula for women with irregular or painful menstrual cycles.

Ingredients

- ✓ 8 1/2 oz. vitex
- ✓ 3/4 oz. dong quai
- ✓ 3/4 oz. licorice
- ✓ 3/4 oz. ginger
- ✓ Cinnamon and orange peel as desired
- ✓ Pinch of cayenne for warmth and flavor (optional)

Directions

1. To make blend: Combine dried herbs; mix well. Store in tightly sealed glass jar. (Dried blend will keep for up to a year.)
2. To make 1 quart tea: Add 8 teaspoons blend to 1 quart cold water in saucepan. Place over low heat; slowly bring to a boil. Cover and simmer for 15 to 20 minutes. Remove

from heat and strain. Sweeten with honey if desired. Drink 3 to 4 cups daily.

Iced Tea

* *

Almond Tea

"This beverage is a wonderful Summer treat that pleases all! Great for parties or just to have on hand."
***Servings**: 16 | **Prep**: 15 m | **Ready In**: 15 m*

Ingredients

- ✓ 3 tablespoons instant iced tea powder
- ✓ 1 cup white sugar
- ✓ 2 cups boiling water
- ✓ 1 (12 ounce) can frozen lemonade concentrate
- ✓ 2 teaspoons vanilla extract
- ✓ 1 tablespoon almond extract

Directions

- ✓ In a 1 gallon container, mix together the instant tea powder and sugar. Pour in the boiling water and lemonade concentrate, and mix well. Stir in the vanilla and almond extracts. Fill container the rest of the way with cold water. Stir and serve over ice, or refrigerate until ready to serve.

Nutritional Information

- ✓ Calories: 103 kcal 5%
- ✓ Fat: 0.1 g < 1%
- ✓ Carbs: 25.7g 8%
- ✓ Protein: 0.2 g < 1%
- ✓ Cholesterol: 0 mg 0%
- ✓ Sodium: 2 mg < 1%

Arnold Palmer

"Named after the golfer, it is said to be his favorite beverage."
***Servings**: 1 | **Prep**: 5 m | **Ready In**: 5 m*

Ingredients
- ✓ 1/3 cup iced tea
- ✓ 1/3 cup prepared lemonade

Directions
- ✓ Pour the iced tea and lemonade into an ice-filled glass; stir to mix.

Nutritional Information
- ✓ Calories: 34 kcal 2%
- ✓ Fat: 0 g < 1%
- ✓ Carbs: 8.9g 3%
- ✓ Protein: 0.1 g < 1%
- ✓ Cholesterol: 0 mg 0%
- ✓ Sodium: 6 mg < 1%

Beverage Cubes

"Everyone has a favorite drink that is always in the fridge...but don't you hate it when your ice cubes melt and make your drink watery? Here's a simple solution! Use your favorite non-carbonated beverage; fruit juice, coffee and prepared drink mix all work great."
***Servings**: 12 | **Prep**: 1 m | **Ready In**: 1 m*

Ingredients
- ✓ 2 cups brewed black tea, cold

Directions

- ✓ Pour the cold tea into an ice cube tray and freeze. Pop out a few whenever you're ready for a tall cool drink.

Nutritional Information

- ✓ Calories: < 1 kcal < 1%
- ✓ Fat: 0 g < 1%
- ✓ Carbs: 0.1g < 1%
- ✓ Protein: 0 g 0%
- ✓ Cholesterol: 0 mg 0%
- ✓ Sodium: 1 mg < 1%

Blueberry-Green Tea Slushie

Blueberries blended with green tea in ice cubes make this a healthy and tasty slushy.

Servings: 4

Ingredients

- ✓ 2 1/2 cups water
- ✓ 3 green tea bags
- ✓ 1 cup blueberries
- ✓ 2 tablespoons agave syrup

Directions

- ✓ Bring 2 cups water to a boil. Add green tea bags and let steep for 5 minutes. Remove tea bags. Divide blueberries between the compartments of an ice cube tray. Cover with tea and freeze. Puree in a blender with remaining tea (1 1/2 cups), 1/2 cup water, and agave syrup. Serve garnished with more berries.

Boston Iced Tea

"After tasting Boston Iced Tea, I just had to try and concoct my own.
Delicious and refreshing! You can also serve with a slice of fresh orange."
***Servings**: 14 | **Prep**: 20 m | **Cook**: 15 m | **Ready In**: 35 m*

Ingredients

- ✓ 1 gallon water
- ✓ 1 cup white sugar
- ✓ 15 tea bags
- ✓ 1 (12 fluid ounce) can frozen cranberry juice concentrate

Directions

- ✓ Put water in large pot, and heat on high until boiling. Add sugar and stir until dissolved. Add teabags and let steep until desired strength is acquired. Stir in cranberry juice concentrate, and allow to cool.

Nutritional Information

- ✓ Calories: 118 kcal 6%
- ✓ Fat: 0 g 0%
- ✓ Carbs: 30.3g 10%
- ✓ Protein: 0 g < 1%
- ✓ Cholesterol: 0 mg 0%
- ✓ Sodium: 9 mg < 1%

Chai Tea Latte

"This is really similar to the brand Oregon® Chai. Simply delicious either
hot or iced! This will save you more money than buying the chai. In India,
each family has their own way of making it, so you should experiment to
find your favorite blend."
***Servings**: 1 | **Prep**: 5 m | **Ready In**: 5 m*

Ingredients

- ✓ 3/4 cup boiling water
- ✓ 1 chai tea bag
- ✓ 1 1/2 teaspoons honey
- ✓ 1 teaspoon white sugar
- ✓ 3/4 cup milk

Directions

1. Pour boiling water over tea bag in a mug; let steep 4 to 6 minutes. Remove and discard tea bag.
2. Stir honey and sugar into tea to dissolve. Stir milk through tea to serve.

Nutritional Information

- ✓ Calories: 145 kcal 7%
- ✓ Fat: 3.6 g 6%
- ✓ Carbs: 22.6g 7%
- ✓ Protein: 6.1 g 12%
- ✓ Cholesterol: 15 mg 5%
- ✓ Sodium: 81 mg 3%

Detox Iced Green Tea

It is time to give your detox drink a twist of tea. The ancient Chinese tea leaves are one of the planets leading sources of antioxidants, so they are sure to flush all poisons from the system right away.

***Servings**: 1 | **Prep**: 5 m*

Ingredients

- ✓ 1 green tea bag or Keurig® cup
- ✓ 1 slice lemon
- ✓ 1 tsp honey or stevia
- ✓ 2 strawberries, sliced
- ✓ 2 slices cucumber

Directions

1. Using either a Keurig® Brewer and green tea K-cup or a green tea bag and boiling water, brew 8-10 fluid ounces of water to make green tea.
2. Chill green tea in refrigerator for 5 minutes. Add cucumber, lemon, strawberries and honey or stevia.
3. Stir to mix ingredients and add ice if desired.
4. Drink daily as a natural detox to rid your body of toxins and for healthy digestion.

Fresh Cranberry Spiced Tea

"A lovely clear red, hot beverage for holiday parties, an afternoon break, for dinner or bedtime as it contains no caffeine. I have been making this for decades and keep it in the fridge all winter. One of my most requested recipes!"

***Servings**: 16 | **Prep**: 10 m | **Cook**: 30 m | **Ready In**: 8 h 40 m*

Ingredients

- ✓ 1 pound fresh or frozen cranberries
- ✓ 3 quarts cold water
- ✓ 2 cups orange juice
- ✓ 2 1/8 cups pineapple juice
- ✓ 1/4 cup lemon juice
- ✓ 2 cups white sugar, or to taste
- ✓ 1 (3 inch) cinnamon stick
- ✓ 1 teaspoon whole cloves
- ✓ 1/2 teaspoon whole allspice berries

Directions

1. Place the cranberries and water into a large pot. Bring to a boil and cook just until the berries pop, about 5

minutes. Remove from the heat and let stand at room temperature until cold, several hours.

2. Strain out the cranberries and stir the orange juice, pineapple juice, lemon juice and sugar into the liquid. Add the cinnamon stick, whole cloves and allspice berries. Bring to a low boil. It is ready to serve at this point, but it is even better if you allow it to sit overnight.

Nutritional Information
- ✓ Calories: 143 kcal 7%
- ✓ Fat: 0.2 g < 1%
- ✓ Carbs: 36.6g 12%
- ✓ Protein: 0.5 g < 1%
- ✓ Cholesterol: 0 mg 0%
- ✓ Sodium: 7 mg < 1%

Friendship Tea

"This is a lemony spiced tea mix with cinnamon and clove that makes great gifts during the holidays, or any time!"
***Servings**: 40 | **Prep**: 10 m | **Ready In**: 10 m*

Ingredients
- ✓ 1/2 cup instant tea powder
- ✓ 1 cup sweetened lemonade powder
- ✓ 1 cup orange-flavored drink mix (e.g. Tang)
- ✓ 1 teaspoon ground cinnamon
- ✓ 1/2 teaspoon ground cloves

Directions
1. In a large bowl, combine instant tea, lemonade powder, orange drink mix, cinnamon and clove. Mix well and store in an airtight container.

2. To serve, Put 2 to 3 teaspoons of mix in a mug. Stir in 1 cup of boiling water. Adjust to taste.

Nutritional Information

- ✓ Calories: 39 kcal 2%
- ✓ Fat: 0 g < 1%
- ✓ Carbs: 9.9g 3%
- ✓ Protein: 0.1 g < 1%
- ✓ Cholesterol: 0 mg 0%
- ✓ Sodium: 2 mg < 1%

Good Ol' Alabama Sweet Tea

"This sweet tea is found in houses, churches, and cafes all over the great state of Alabama. If you're north of the Mason-Dixon, you've NEVER had tea this good! Fresh-squeezed lemon, lime, or orange juice can be added for an extra flavor."

Servings: 16 | **Prep**: 1 m | **Cook**: 10 m | **Ready In**: 11 m

Ingredients

- ✓ 2 cups sugar
- ✓ 1/2 gallon water
- ✓ 1 tray ice cubes
- ✓ 3 family sized teabags of orange pekoe tea
- ✓ 3 cups cold water, or as needed

Directions

1. Pour the sugar into a large pitcher. Bring water to a boil in a large pan. When the water begins to boil, remove from the heat, and place the teabags in. Let steep for 5 to 6 minutes.

2. Remove tea bags, and return tea to the heat. Bring just to a boil, then pour into the pitcher, and stir until the sugar is dissolved. Fill the pitcher half way with ice, and stir

until most of it melts. Then fill the pitcher the rest of the way with cold water, and stir until blended.

Nutritional Information

- ✓ Calories: 97 kcal 5%
- ✓ Fat: 0 g 0%
- ✓ Carbs: 25g 8%
- ✓ Protein: 0 g 0%
- ✓ Cholesterol: 0 mg 0%
- ✓ Sodium: 4 mg < 1%

Green Tea Berry Delight

"This refreshing treat is as healthy as it is beautiful! It's packed with antioxidants and a great alternative to that calorie laden latte!"
Servings: 1 | **Prep**: 5 m | **Ready In**: 5 m

Ingredients

- ✓ 1/2 cup frozen blueberries
- ✓ 4 frozen strawberries
- ✓ 2 cups iced green tea

Directions

- ✓ Place the blueberries and strawberries in the bottom of a tall glass. Pour the green tea over the berries.

Nutritional Information

- ✓ Calories: 59 kcal 3%
- ✓ Fat: 0.6 g < 1%
- ✓ Carbs: 14.7g 5%
- ✓ Protein: 0.5 g 1%
- ✓ Cholesterol: 0 mg 0%
- ✓ Sodium: 16 mg < 1%

Hawaiian Plantation Iced Tea

"I first tasted this tea in a popular Italian restaurant in my college hometown of Kailua. I have been craving it ever since, and have experimented with a few proportions. Add more tea leaves for a stronger tea, but do not steep longer or the tea will end up tasting bitter. (If it does, add a pinch of baking soda.) Always make something to your liking! This is also great to serve at showers."

Servings: *8* | ***Prep***: *10 m* | ***Ready In***: *1 h 40 m*

Ingredients

- ✓ 1 quart barely boiling hot water
- ✓ 4 orange pekoe tea bags
- ✓ 1 quart ice cold water
- ✓ 1 (16 ounce) can pineapple juice
- ✓ 1/2 cup simple syrup (optional)
- ✓ 1 fresh pineapple - peeled, cored, and cut into spears

Directions

1. Pour the barely boiling hot water into a large pitcher, and add the tea bags. Steep the tea 2 to 4 minutes. Remove the tea bags, and pour in the ice water. Pour in the pineapple juice. Refrigerate until thoroughly chilled, about 1 1/2 hours.

2. Pour the tea over ice, garnish with pineapple spears, and serve.

Nutritional Information

- ✓ Calories: 152 kcal 8%
- ✓ Fat: 0.3 g < 1%
- ✓ Carbs: 39.3g 13%
- ✓ Protein: 1.1 g 2%
- ✓ Cholesterol: 0 mg 0%
- ✓ Sodium: 10 mg < 1%

Hibiscus Iced Tea Sparkler

Hibiscus Iced Tea Sparkler is a very refreshing and delicious spring or summer-drink made with hibiscus tea and sparkling water.
Servings*: 6 - 8 |* ***Prep****: 10 m |* ***Total Time****: 1 h 30 m*

Ingredients

- ✓ 4 cups boiling water
- ✓ 8 hibiscus tea bags
- ✓ 1/2 cup honey
- ✓ Ice
- ✓ 2 cups sparkling water (I use Perrier)
- ✓ 1/4 cup mint leaves, for garnish
- ✓ Strawberries, for garnish

Directions

1. In a large pitcher, combine tea bags, honey, and boiling water; let steep 30 minutes to 1 hour, depending on how strong you like your tea.
2. Remove tea bags.
3. Add ice to pitcher and stir in sparkling water.
4. Add mint.
5. Refrigerate for 1 hour or until chilled.
6. Garnish with strawberries.
7. Serve.

Honey Lemon Tea

"This is my favorite tea, my dad used to make it for me all the time. It is a sweet and sour tea. You taste the honey and then the lemon! YUM,YUM,YUM! Great for soothing sore throats!"
Servings*: 1 |* ***Prep****: 1 m |* ***Cook****: 2 m |* ***Ready In****: 10 m*

Ingredients

- ✓ 1 cup water
- ✓ 2 teaspoons honey
- ✓ 1 teaspoon fresh lemon juice
- ✓ 1 teaspoon white sugar, or to taste

Directions

- ✓ Pour water into a mug. Add honey and heat in the microwave for 1 minute and 30 seconds. Stir in lemon juice, mixing until honey is dissolved, then stir in the sugar.

Nutritional Information

- ✓ Calories: 63 kcal 3%
- ✓ Fat: 0 g 0%
- ✓ Carbs: 16.9g 5%
- ✓ Protein: 0.1 g < 1%
- ✓ Cholesterol: 0 mg 0%
- ✓ Sodium: < 1 mg < 1%

Honey Milk Tea - Hong Kong Style

"I came up with this recipe after reading many Chinese posts; none of them sounded like the milk tea I have had before. Honey milk tea is what I always order when I go to a tea place. Technically, bubble tea is not much different from milk tea (I am not sure why they separate them into two different categories in the tea shop). There are also different styles of bubble/milk tea, like Hong Kong style, Taiwan style, etc. This is a Hong Kong-style milk tea."

*Servings: 1 | **Prep**: 5 m | **Ready In**: 15 m*

Ingredients

- ✓ 2 orange pekoe tea bags
- ✓ 1 cup boiling water

- ✓ 5 ice cubes
- ✓ 4 teaspoons sweetened condensed milk
- ✓ 3 teaspoons honey

Directions

1. Steep the tea bags in hot water until the color turns dark red, about 3 to 5 minutes. Discard the tea bags and let the tea cool.

2. Combine the ice cubes, sweetened condensed milk, and honey in a glass or cocktail shaker. Pour in the tea and mix well. (If the tea is still warm, the ice may melt; add more ice if desired.) A strong, flavorful milk tea is ready for you to enjoy.

Cook's Note

- ✓ A good strong-flavored tea is the key to making good milk tea. Add more honey to taste if you like a sweeter tea. If you have a martini shaker, you may use it to mix the milk tea.

Nutritional Information

- ✓ Calories: 151 kcal 8%
- ✓ Fat: 2.2 g 3%
- ✓ Carbs: 32.4g 10%
- ✓ Protein: 2.1 g 4%
- ✓ Cholesterol: 9 mg 3%
- ✓ Sodium: 44 mg 2%

Iced Green Tea Citrus Detox Drink

Ingredients

- ✓ Lime - 1 (sliced)
- ✓ Lemon - 1 (sliced)
- ✓ Orange - 1 (sliced)

- ✓ Green Tea - 4 teaspoons
- ✓ Basil leaves/tulsi - ¼ cup
- ✓ Water - 10 glasses

Directions

1. Brew green tea in 2 glass of water. Let it cool down and strain it.
2. Add remaining glasses of water, brewed green tea, lemon slices, basil leaves, lime slices, orange slices in a glass jar and mix well.
3. Close the jar and refrigerate for minimum 4 hours.
4. Strain the infused water, pour in serving glass with ice-cubes and enjoy.

Iced Tea II

"This iced tea is fabulous - it tastes like the brand names!"
Servings: 8 | **Prep**: 10 m | **Cook**: 1 h | **Ready In**: 1 h 10 m

Ingredients

- ✓ 8 cups water
- ✓ 3 orange pekoe tea bags
- ✓ 3/4 cup white sugar
- ✓ 1/2 cup lemon juice

Directions

1. In a large saucepan, heat water to a rapid boil. Remove from heat and drop in the tea bags. Cover and let steep for 1 hour.
2. In a large pitcher, combine the steeped tea and the sugar. Stir until sugar is dissolved, then stir in lemon juice. Refrigerate until chilled.

Nutritional Information

- ✓ Calories: 76 kcal 4%

- ✓ Fat: 0 g 0%
- ✓ Carbs: 20.1g 6%
- ✓ Protein: 0.1 g < 1%
- ✓ Cholesterol: 0 mg 0%
- ✓ Sodium: < 1 mg < 1%

Iced Tea III

"Cool, refreshing, and abundant summer drink. Serve in a tall glass over ice."

***Servings**: 16 | **Prep**: 10 m | **Ready In**: 2 h 10 m*

Ingredients

- ✓ 6 black tea bags
- ✓ 1/2 cup white sugar
- ✓ 1 gallon boiling water
- ✓ 1 (6 ounce) can frozen lemonade concentrate

Directions

- ✓ Place the tea bags and sugar into a 1 gallon glass jar. Fill with boiling water. Let steep for 2 hours at room temperature. Remove and discard tea bags. Stir in lemonade concentrate. Refrigerate until cool.

Nutritional Information

- ✓ Calories: 49 kcal 2%
- ✓ Fat: 0 g < 1%
- ✓ Carbs: 12.7g 4%
- ✓ Protein: 0 g < 1%
- ✓ Cholesterol: 0 mg 0%
- ✓ Sodium: 8 mg < 1%

Iced Turmeric Green Tea

Ingredients

- ✓ 2 cups (500ml) water
- ✓ 1 inch fresh ginger root, minced
- ✓ 2 teaspoons ground turmeric (or 1 inch fresh turmeric root)
- ✓ 1 green tea bag
- ✓ 1 pinch of salt
- ✓ 1/4 cup (85g) honey
- ✓ Ice and fresh lime slices to serve (optional)

Directions

1. In a medium pot, bring water close to a boil and add minced ginger, turmeric, honey, and salt. Simmer for 10 minutes then turn off the heat. Add the green tea bag and steep for 3 minutes, then take out. Strain out the solids using a fine mesh strainer and set aside.
2. Pick any sized glass or mason jar you like, fill 3/4 height with ice cube, pour the tea over the ice. Add fresh lime juice, honey to taste, garnish with a slice of lime, and enjoy!

Instant Russian Tea

"This recipe was given to me two Christmas's ago from a very good friend. She said to pass it on. So I am."
***Servings:** 100 | **Prep:** 10 m | **Ready In:** 10 m*

Ingredients

- ✓ 2 cups orange-flavored drink mix (e.g. Tang)
- ✓ 2 cups white sugar
- ✓ 1/4 cup instant tea powder

- ✓ 3/4 cup lemon-flavored instant tea powder
- ✓ 1 teaspoon ground cinnamon
- ✓ 1 teaspoon ground cloves

Directions

1. In a large bowl, combine orange drink mix, sugar, tea powder, cinnamon and cloves. Mix well and store in an airtight container.
2. To serve, put 3 teaspoons of mix in a mug. Stir in 1 cup boiling water. Adjust to taste.

Nutritional Information

- ✓ Calories: 32 kcal 2%
- ✓ Fat: 0 g < 1%
- ✓ Carbs: 8.4g 3%
- ✓ Protein: 0.1 g < 1%
- ✓ Cholesterol: 0 mg 0%
- ✓ Sodium: < 1 mg < 1%

Jasmine Tea Tangerineade

The clink-clink of ice in an Arnold Palmer -- the drink that joins our two national summer refreshments, lemonade and iced tea -- can be heard anywhere from backyard barbecues to beach picnics. This not-so-standard rendition includes Jasmine-tea pearls, which bestow floral notes on sweet tangerine juice.

Servings: *8 |* **Yield:** *Makes 7 1/2 Cups*

Ingredients

- ✓ 3 1/4 cups water
- ✓ 3 tablespoons jasmine pearls
- ✓ 1 1/4 cups Simple Syrup
- ✓ 3 cups fresh tangerine juice, strained (from 8 to 10 tangerines)

Directions

1. Bring water to a simmer in a small saucepan. Remove from heat, add jasmine pearls, and infuse for 2 1/2 minutes. Strain through a small sieve into a pitcher. Discard pearls. Let cool.

2. Add syrup and tangerine juice to pitcher. Divide tangerineade among ice-filled glasses. (Or cover, and refrigerate for up to 3 days.)

Lemon Almond Tea

"This tea is very refreshing on hot summer days. You can adjust it by decreasing the sugar, or increasing the almond."
Servings: 12 | **Prep**: 15 m | **Cook**: 15 m | **Ready In**: 30 m

Ingredients

- ✓ 2 family size black tea bags
- ✓ 4 cups boiling water
- ✓ 2 lemons, thinly sliced
- ✓ 1 cup sugar
- ✓ 1 tablespoon almond extract
- ✓ 2 teaspoons vanilla extract
- ✓ 1 (2 liter) bottle lemon-lime flavored carbonated beverage, chilled

Directions

1. In a saucepan, brew tea bags in hot water for 15 minutes. While waiting for tea to brew, squeeze the lemon slices as you put them into a large pitcher. Pour in sugar.

2. Pour brewed tea into the pitcher with the sugar and lemons. You can let this sit in refrigerator for up to 1 day, or use it right away. When ready to serve, stir in almond extract, vanilla extract and lemon lime soda.

Nutritional Information

- ✓ Calories: 142 kcal 7%
- ✓ Fat: 0.1 g < 1%
- ✓ Carbs: 36.7g 12%
- ✓ Protein: 0.2 g < 1%
- ✓ Cholesterol: 0 mg 0%
- ✓ Sodium: 20 mg < 1%

Lemonade-Mint Iced Tea

"A refreshing and easy to prepare iced tea. You can vary the amounts of mint and sugar depending on your tastes."

Servings: 12 | **Prep**: 25 m | **Ready In**: 25 m

Ingredients

- ✓ 3 tablespoons crushed fresh mint leaves
- ✓ 1 quart boiling water
- ✓ 1/2 cup instant iced tea powder
- ✓ 1 cup white sugar
- ✓ 2 quarts cold water
- ✓ 1 (6 ounce) can frozen lemonade concentrate, thawed

Directions

1. In a 1 gallon pitcher, combine the mint leaves, 1 quart of boiling water, instant tea powder and sugar. Stir to dissolve sugar. Let stand for 15 minutes.
2. Stir in the cold water and lemonade concentrate. Serve in tall glasses over ice. Strain out mint leaves, if desired.

Nutritional Information

- ✓ Calories: 102 kcal 5%
- ✓ Fat: 0 g < 1%
- ✓ Carbs: 26.1g 8%
- ✓ Protein: 0.3 g < 1%

✓ Cholesterol: 0 mg 0%

✓ Sodium: 9 mg < 1%

Licorice Mint Iced Tea

Peppermint ranks high among America's favorite types of mint tea, but you can substitute equal amounts of any variety for this recipe.
***Servings**: 4 | **Prep Time**: 5 mins| **Total Time**: 30 mins*

Ingredients

✓ 2 1/2 teaspoons dried licorice root

✓ 1 cinnamon stick

✓ 1/2 cup dried peppermint leaves

✓ 1/2 cup raw honey

✓ 4 sprigs of fresh mint (optional)

Directions

1. In a large pot bring 6 cups of water to a boil over high heat. Stir in the licorice and cinnamon; lower to a simmer, partially cover the pot, and simmer for 10 minutes. Remove from heat, stir in peppermint, cover, and steep for 10 minutes.

2. Meanwhile, place a large strainer lined with cheesecloth or a damp paper towel over another pot or heatproof bowl. Strain tea, pressing on herbs to extract all liquid. Stir in honey until dissolved and let cool completely, about 1 hour. Fill four tall glasses with ice. Pour tea over ice and garnish each glass with a mint sprig, if desired. Serve immediately.

Peach Iced Tea

Peaches and blackberries sweeten iced tea.
***Servings:** 8*

Ingredients

- ✓ 2 black-tea bags, such as English breakfast
- ✓ 8 cups boiling water
- ✓ 4 peaches
- ✓ 1/4 cup sugar
- ✓ 1/2 cup peach nectar
- ✓ Blackberries, for garnish

Directions

1. Put tea bags and the boiling water in a medium saucepan or heatproof bowl. Let stand 5 minutes. Discard tea bags. Transfer tea to a large pitcher.

2. Cut 2 of the peaches into 8 wedges each. Add sliced peaches and the sugar to the tea. Stir tea until sugar has dissolved. Let cool completely.

3. Stir in peach nectar. Refrigerate tea until cold (or up to 1 week in an airtight container). Just before serving, remove peaches; discard. Cut remaining peaches into 8 wedges each. Add peaches and blackberries to the tea. Serve over ice.

Iced Tea

"This is a peach- and orange-flavored iced tea, great on a hot summer day. A nectarine can be substituted for the peach. A mandarin orange can be substituted for the clementine."

***Servings:** 8 | **Prep:** 10 m | **Ready In:** 1 h 10 m*

Ingredients

- ✓ 1 large fresh peach, sliced

- ✓ 1 clementine, peeled and segmented
- ✓ 1 tablespoon white sugar, or to taste
- ✓ 8 cups boiling water
- ✓ 4 Earl Grey tea bags

Directions

- ✓ Place peach, clementine, and sugar in a pitcher. Mash the fruit using a spoon; add water and tea bags and stir. Refrigerate until cool, about 1 hour. Remove fruit and tea bags using a slotted spoon.

Nutritional Information

- ✓ Calories: 15 kcal < 1%
- ✓ Fat: 0 g < 1%
- ✓ Carbs: 3.7g 1%
- ✓ Protein: 0.1 g < 1%
- ✓ Cholesterol: 0 mg 0%
- ✓ Sodium: 8 mg < 1%

Peach Tea

"This is a very light peach tea, great for a summer day."
Servings: 10 | **Prep**: 5 m | **Cook**: 15 m | **Ready In**: 20 m

Ingredients

- ✓ 3 cups water
- ✓ 3 family size tea bags
- ✓ 2 fresh peaches - peeled, pitted, and sliced
- ✓ 1 cup water
- ✓ 1 1/2 teaspoons stevia powder

Directions

1. Bring 3 cups water to a boil in a saucepan over high heat. Add the tea bags, and steep for 15 minutes. Remove tea bags.

2. Meanwhile, place peaches with 1 cup water into the jar of a blender, and blend until very smooth. Pour the peach mixture, tea, and stevia powder into a 1 gallon pitcher. Fill the pitcher to the top with water, and stir until blended.

Nutritional Information
- ✓ Calories: 5 kcal < 1%
- ✓ Fat: 0 g 0%
- ✓ Carbs: 1.6g < 1%
- ✓ Protein: 0 g < 1%
- ✓ Cholesterol: 0 mg 0%
- ✓ Sodium: < 1 mg < 1%

Randy's Texas Tea

"On a hot day in Texas, nothing is more refreshing than this sweet, fruity, non-alcoholic summer iced tea."

***Servings:** 8 | **Prep:** 10 m | **Ready In:** 10 m*

Ingredients
- ✓ 1 cup white sugar
- ✓ 1/4 teaspoon salt
- ✓ 1 cup hot water
- ✓ 6 cups brewed black tea, cold
- ✓ 2 cups orange juice
- ✓ 1/2 cup lemon juice
- ✓ 1 orange, sliced into rounds
- ✓ 1 lemon, sliced into rounds
- ✓ 1 lime, sliced into rounds

Directions
- ✓ In a large pitcher, combine sugar, salt and hot water. Stir until completely dissolved. Sir in the tea, orange juice and

lemon juice. Serve in tall glasses with ice and slices of citrus fruit.

Nutritional Information

- ✓ Calories: 145 kcal 7%
- ✓ Fat: 0.2 g < 1%
- ✓ Carbs: 38.1g 12%
- ✓ Protein: 0.9 g 2%
- ✓ Cholesterol: 0 mg 0%
- ✓ Sodium: 79 mg 3%

Raspberry Iced Tea

"This is the best, easiest summer drink EVER!"
Servings: 10 | Prep: 5 m | Cook: 10 m | Ready In: 25 m

Ingredients

- ✓ 1 gallon water
- ✓ 3 (3 ounce) gallon-size tea bags
- ✓ 1 cup fresh raspberries
- ✓ 1/2 cup white sugar
- ✓ 1/2 cup powdered lemonade mix (such as Country Time®)
- ✓ Ice cubes

Directions

- ✓ Bring the water to a boil in a large pot, and stir in the tea bags, raspberries, and sugar until the sugar has dissolved. Allow the mixture to steep until the desired level of tea flavor is reached, 3 to 5 minutes; remove tea bags, and stir in the lemonade mix until dissolved. Pour tea into pitchers, and add ice to cool.

Nutritional Information

- ✓ Calories: 86 kcal 4%

- ✓ Fat: 0.1 g < 1%
- ✓ Carbs: 22.2g 7%
- ✓ Protein: 0.1 g < 1%
- ✓ Cholesterol: 0 mg 0%
- ✓ Sodium: 15 mg < 1%

Raspberry Rosehip Iced Tea

Fruit juice is a great way to sweeten iced tea brews naturally. The raisins in this recipe also add a natural sweetness.
***Servings**: 4 | **Prep**: 5 m | **Total Time**: 30 m*

Ingredients

- ✓ 1/4 cup dried rosehips
- ✓ 1/2 cup raisins
- ✓ 1/2 cup dried raspberry leaves
- ✓ 1 1/2 cups naturally sweetened raspberry or cherry juice
- ✓ 1/3 cup fresh orange juice
- ✓ 4 orange slices, for garnish (optional)

Directions

1. In a large pot bring 4 1/2 cups of water to a boil over high heat. Stir in the rosehips and raisins. Partially cover the pot, lower the heat, and simmer for 10 minutes. Remove pot from heat, stir in raspberry leaves, cover, and steep for 10 minutes.

2. Meanwhile, place a large strainer lined with cheesecloth or a damp paper towel over another pot or heatproof bowl. Strain tea, pressing on the herbs to extract all liquid. Add raspberry and orange juices and stir to blend. Let brew cool completely, about 45 minutes. Fill four tall glasses with ice. Pour tea over ice and garnish each with an orange slice, if desired. Serve immediately.

Smooth Sweet Tea

"Southern sweet tea, perfect for hot summer days!"
Servings: *8* | ***Prep***: *5 m* | ***Cook***: *15 m* | ***Ready In***: *3 h 20 m*

Ingredients

- ✓ 1 pinch baking soda
- ✓ 2 cups boiling water
- ✓ 6 tea bags
- ✓ 3/4 cup white sugar
- ✓ 6 cups cool water

Directions

1. Sprinkle a pinch of baking soda into a 64-ounce, heat-proof, glass pitcher. Pour in boiling water, and add tea bags. Cover, and allow to steep for 15 minutes.
2. Remove tea bags, and discard; stir in sugar until dissolved. Pour in cool water, then refrigerate until cold.

Nutritional Information

- ✓ Calories: 73 kcal 4%
- ✓ Fat: 0 g 0%
- ✓ Carbs: 18.7g 6%
- ✓ Protein: 0 g 0%
- ✓ Cholesterol: 0 mg 0%
- ✓ Sodium: 41 mg 2%

South Carolina Sweet Tea

"Remember, this is the south where simplicity is the secret to most recipes. Follow this to the 'T' and you will have sweet tea, Sand Lapper (South Carolina) style."

*Servings: 16 | **Prep**: 1 m | **Cook**: 10 m | **Ready In**: 11 m*

Ingredients

- ✓ 3 family size tea bags
- ✓ 2 cups white sugar

Directions

- ✓ Using an electric coffee maker, Place the 3 tea bags in the strainer basket (not in the pot). Brew the tea as you would coffee. Pour the sugar in a gallon pitcher. Pour in the hot tea. Continue to run coffee maker with the tea bags until you have enough tea to fill the pitcher. Allow to cool completely at room temperature, then refrigerate.

Nutritional Information

- ✓ Calories: 97 kcal 5%
- ✓ Fat: 0 g 0%
- ✓ Carbs: 25g 8%
- ✓ Protein: 0 g 0%
- ✓ Cholesterol: 0 mg 0%
- ✓ Sodium: 0 mg 0%

Stamina Tea

Instead of relying on lots of caffeine to keep you alert and energetic, try our homemade herbal chai to build your body's reserves.
***Yield**: Makes 1 Quart*

Ingredients

- ✓ 3 teaspoons dried eleuthero
- ✓ 2 teaspoons dried burdock root
- ✓ 2 teaspoons dried licorice root
- ✓ 1 teaspoon dried (or 2 teaspoons fresh chopped) ginger
- ✓ 1 teaspoon cinnamon chips (or 1 cinnamon stick)

✓ 1 teaspoon cardamom pods

Directions

✓ Simmer herbs in 1 quart of water for 20 minutes. Strain and discard herbs. Pour a cup, adding milk and honey to taste if desired. Keep remaining tea in a jar or thermos. Tea will keep for two days in refrigerator.

Sweet Lime Iced Tea

"What's more Southern than sweet iced tea? I've lived in Florida all my life, yet I'm not a huge fan of the overly sweet iced tea that is popular here in the South. My grandma has made this version for as long as I can remember and it is the BEST!! Not too sweet, and not too bitter...and the fresh lime juice --- amazing!!!"

Servings: 16 | *Prep*: 10 m | *Cook*: 5 m | *Ready In*: 4 h

Ingredients

✓ 1 gallon boiling water
✓ 6 black tea bags
✓ 1 1/2 cups white sugar
✓ 4 limes, juiced

Directions

✓ Pour the water into a gallon sized jar over the tea bags. Allow to steep for 45 minutes. Remove and discard the tea bags. Stir in the sugar and lime juice until the sugar has dissolved. Cool to room temperature; refrigerate until cold before serving.

Nutritional Information

✓ Calories: 75 kcal 4%
✓ Fat: 0 g < 1%
✓ Carbs: 19.5g 6%
✓ Protein: 0 g < 1%

✓ Cholesterol: 0 mg 0%

✓ Sodium: 7 mg < 1%

The Best Lemon Iced Tea

"This is the best iced tea I've ever tasted. It comes very close to the Good Host® brand we Canadians are used to."
Servings: *16* | **Prep**: *5 m* | **Ready In**: *1 h 5 m*

Ingredients

- 4 green tea bags
- 4 orange pekoe tea bags
- 6 cups boiling water
- 1 cup white sugar
- 1 (12 ounce) can frozen lemonade concentrate
- 1/2 lemon, juiced
- Cold water, or as needed

Directions

1. Place green tea bags and black tea bags in a 1-gallon glass jar. Pour boiling water over tea bags; steep for 30 minutes.

2. Remove tea bags; stir in sugar and lemonade concentrate until dissolved. Fill jar to the top with cold water; stir in lemon juice. Chill in the refrigerator until cold. Serve over ice.

Nutritional Information

✓ Calories: 99 kcal 5%

✓ Fat: 0.1 g < 1%

✓ Carbs: 25.7g 8%

✓ Protein: 0.1 g < 1%

✓ Cholesterol: 0 mg 0%

✓ Sodium: 4 mg < 1%

Very Popular Bubble Tea

"Bubble tea is very popular, especially to Asians, but now, more and more people from different backgrounds like the taste of it. I'm no expert at this, but I do know Directions it. It's simple but some of the ingredients may be a little tough to find. Just be patient and look for them in Chinese grocery stores. It is worth the trouble!"

Servings: *1* | **Prep**: *10 m* | **Cook**: *20 m* | **Ready In**: *1 h 30 m*

Ingredients

- ✓ 1 teaspoon white sugar
- ✓ 1/3 cup pearl tapioca
- ✓ 1 cup brewed black tea
- ✓ 2 tablespoons milk
- ✓ 4 teaspoons white sugar
- ✓ 1 cup ice cubes

Directions

1. In a small saucepan, bring 2 cups water to a boil. Stir in 1 teaspoon sugar until it dissolves. Toss in the pearl tapioca. Cook for about 20 minutes. Rinse, drain, and refrigerate until chilled.

2. Pour tea, milk, and 4 teaspoons sugar into a cocktail shaker. Stir until the sugar has dissolved and the milk is well mixed in. Add the ice cubes, and shake so the whole drink can get cold. Pour into a glass, and add tapioca.

Notes

- ✓ This drink can be turned into Bubble Green Tea if you use green tea instead.
- ✓ If you can find it, use Chinese rock sugar, or bing tong, to cook the tapioca with.

Nutritional Information

- ✓ Calories: 280 kcal 14%
- ✓ Fat: 0.6 g < 1%
- ✓ Carbs: 67.9g 22%
- ✓ Protein: 1.1 g 2%
- ✓ Cholesterol: 2 mg < 1%
- ✓ Sodium: 27 mg 1%

Watermelon Green Tea Detox Water

Ingredients

- ✓ Watermelon - 1 cup (cubed)
- ✓ Green Tea - 2 teaspoons
- ✓ Lemon - 1 (thinly sliced)
- ✓ Mint leaves - ½ cup
- ✓ Water - 8 glasses

Directions

1. Brew green tea in 1 glass of water. Let it cool down and strain it.
2. Add remaining glasses of water, brewed green tea, watermelon cubes, mint leaves, lemon slices in a glass jar and mix well.
3. Close the jar and refrigerate for minimum 6 hours.
4. Strain the infused water and enjoy.

Seven: More Healthy Drink

***

Avocado and Mango Milkshake

Drink this delicious shake right away before the avocado oxidizes and turns brown.
Servings: *6*

Ingredients
- ✓ 1 avocado, pitted and peeled
- ✓ 1 mango, peeled, pitted, and coarsely chopped
- ✓ 1 pint low-fat vanilla frozen yogurt
- ✓ 1/2 to 3/4 cup low-fat milk

Directions
- ✓ Combine all of the ingredients in a blender and puree until smooth, adding more milk to thin, if desired.

Blueberry Pomegranate Slushy

This cooler has a nice piquant sweet-tart flavor.
Servings: *1*

Ingredients
- ✓ 1/2 cup frozen blueberries
- ✓ 1/2 cup pomegranate juice
- ✓ 1 teaspoon agave
- ✓ 1/2 cup ice

Directions
- ✓ Puree blueberries, pomegranate juice, agave, and ice in a blender until smooth. Serve immediately.

Cantaloupe Yogurt Drink

Try a cool smoothie like this one on a hot summer morning.
***Servings**: 2*

Ingredients
- ✓ 3 cups cantaloupe chunks (from 1/2 cantaloupe)
- ✓ 2 cups low-fat plain yogurt
- ✓ 2 to 3 tablespoons honey
- ✓ Ice cubes, for serving

Directions
- ✓ In a blender, place cantaloupe, yogurt, and honey. Blend on high speed until smooth. Serve over ice.

Chamomile Cooler

Chamomile and lemon-flavored herbs create a delicate, delightful tea. We used lemon verbena, which lends a pleasantly sweet flavor for a refreshing and light tea.
***Servings**: 4 | **Prep**: 5 mins | **Total time**: 20 mins*

Ingredients
- ✓ 1/2 cup dried chamomile flowers
- ✓ 2 tablespoons dried lemon verbena leaves
- ✓ 1/3 cup raw honey

Directions
1. In a large pot bring 6 cups of water to a boil over high heat. Remove pot from heat and stir in the chamomile and lemon verbena. Cover and steep for 10 minutes.
2. Meanwhile, place a large strainer lined with cheesecloth or a damp paper towel over another pot or heat-proof bowl. Strain tea, pressing on the herbs to extract all

liquid. Stir in honey until it dissolves, and let the tea cool completely, about 1 hour. Fill four tall glasses with ice. Pour tea over ice and serve immediately.

Cinnamon and Spice Hot Cocoa

This cocoa gets extra heat from ancho chile powder, while a touch of cinnamon rounds out the flavor. Serve with marshmallows for a finishing touch.

Servings: *4 |* **Prep Time:** *5 mins|* **Total Time:** *20 mins*

Ingredients
- ✓ 4 cups skim milk
- ✓ 1/2 cup unsweetened cocoa powder
- ✓ 1/2 cup sugar
- ✓ 1/4 teaspoon ground cinnamon
- ✓ 1/2 teaspoon ancho chile powder
- ✓ Coarse salt
- ✓ Marshmallows (optional), for serving

Directions

In a medium pot, whisk together milk, cocoa powder, sugar, cinnamon, chile powder, and pinch of salt over medium-high until combined. Bring to a boil, then reduce heat and simmer 5 minutes. Pour cocoa into four mugs and serve immediately with marshmallows if desired.

Dandelion Tonic

All parts of the dandelion plant are edible and nutritious. Natural sweeteners are helpful in making this tonic taste a little like an old-fashioned root beer.

Yield: *Makes 1 Quart*

Ingredients

- ✓ 2 teaspoons dried raw dandelion root
- ✓ 1 teaspoon dried burdock root
- ✓ 2 teaspoons dried sarsaparilla root
- ✓ 1 teaspoon cinnamon chips
- ✓ 1/2 teaspoon dried gingerroot pieces
- ✓ 1/8 teaspoon dried orange peel
- ✓ Honey or stevia leaf (optional)

Directions

- ✓ Add herbs to 1 quart cold water and bring to a boil. Cover and simmer 15 - 20 minutes. Strain; add honey or stevia to taste. Drink 2 - 4 cups daily.

Fire Cider Tonic

Fend off viruses with zesty herbal vinegar. Try a tablespoon as needed when you're feeling unwell; drizzle on veggies for an immune boost.

Ingredients

- ✓ 1/2 cup chopped ginseng root, fresh or dried
- ✓ 1/4 cup grated ginger root
- ✓ 1/4 cup grated horseradish root
- ✓ 1/8 cup chopped garlic
- ✓ Cayenne pepper
- ✓ Apple cider vinegar
- ✓ Honey

Directions

1. Combine chopped ginseng root, grated ginger root, grated horseradish root, and garlic.

2. Add cayenne to taste. Pour in enough apple cider vinegar to cover the herbs by an inch or two, then seal tightly. Let sit for four weeks.
3. Strain the herbs from the vinegar. Sweeten with honey to taste.

Herbal Stress Release

We cannot make stress disappear, but we can soothe some of the effects with help from a few of nature's simple remedies.
Yield: Makes 1 Quart

Ingredients
- ✓ 2 teaspoons green milky oat tops
- ✓ 2 teaspoons chamomile
- ✓ 2 teaspoons lemon balm
- ✓ 1 teaspoon lavender
- ✓ 1 teaspoon rose petals
- ✓ 1 teaspoon chrysanthemum

Directions
- ✓ Pour 1 quart boiling water over herbs. Cover and steep for at least 15 minutes. Strain and sweeten with stevia or a touch of honey.

Homemade Chai

Our version of the popular spiced tea is more flavorful and far healthier than what you'd get at a coffee house.
Servings: 2

Ingredients

- ✓ 2 green cardamom pods, lightly crushed
- ✓ 1/8 teaspoon black peppercorns
- ✓ 2 cloves
- ✓ 1 cinnamon stick
- ✓ 1 1 1/2-inch piece fresh ginger, peeled and thinly sliced
- ✓ 2 cups water
- ✓ 2 tablespoons brown sugar
- ✓ 2 bags black tea, such as Assam or Darjeeling
- ✓ 3/4 cup reduced-fat milk

Directions

1. Bring spices, ginger, and water to a boil. Reduce to a simmer until liquid becomes aromatic, about 15 minutes. Whisk in sugar, then add tea bags; turn off heat and let steep 3 minutes.

2. While tea is steeping, warm a serving pot by rinsing several times with very hot water. Strain tea mixture through a fine strainer or a coffee filter into pot. Heat milk over medium heat until just simmering. Whisk until frothy. Pour into serving pot, stirring well to combine.

Hot Rice Breakfast Drink

Cooked rice stays fresh for up to seven days and can taste even better the second time around. This recipe was created with flexibility in mind, and is a great way to use up leftover ingredients.

Servings: 4

Ingredients

- ✓ Cooked rice
- ✓ Skim milk (enough to cover rice by about half an inch)
- ✓ Honey to taste

✓ Cinnamon

Directions

✓ Heat cooked rice and skim milk together. Stir in honey to taste, and sprinkle with cinnamon (if desired, take some of the hot milk and whisk briskly to "foam," then pour over top).

Kale Lemonade

Servings: 1 | Prep: 5 mins | Total time: 5 mins

Ingredients

✓ 1 3/4 pounds kale with stems, chopped
✓ 2 apples, such as Honeycrisp, chopped (with peels and cores)
✓ 1 lemon, chopped (with rind and pith)

Directions

✓ Pass kale, apples, and lemon through a juicer. Stir to combine; serve.

Kefir with Berries

Kefir, a fermented-milk drink full of vitamins and beneficial microorganisms, is even better when blended with fresh, organic red and golden rasp- berries or any other fruit that's in season. If you don't have kefir, substitute buttermilk.
Servings: 2

Ingredients

✓ 2 cups nonfat kefir, yogurt, or buttermilk
✓ 1 to 1 1/2 cups berries
✓ 1 tablespoon honey or pure maple syrup (optional)

Directions

✓ Place all ingredients in the jar of a blender. Blend until smooth. Divide evenly between 2 glasses; serve immediately.

Mango Lassi

Instead of serving a heavy milk shake, whip up a refreshing Indian yogurt drink; this one has mangoes and lime juice.
Servings: 6 | **Yield**: *Makes 5 Cups*

Ingredients

✓ 2 ripe mangoes (1 pound each)
✓ 1 cup plain yogurt
✓ 2 tablespoons freshly squeezed lime juice
✓ 2 tablespoons honey
✓ 2 cups small ice cubes

Directions

✓ Peel mangoes, and remove pits; coarsely chop flesh. Puree mangoes and yogurt in a blender until smooth. Add lime juice and honey; pulse to combine. Add ice; blend until incorporated. Serve immediately.

Mulled Apple Cider

Cloves and cinnamon are key to what makes mulled cider so delicious.
Servings: 8 | **Prep**: *10 mins* | **Total time**: *30 mins*

Ingredients

✓ 8 cups apple cider
✓ 2 cinnamon sticks

- ✓ 1 teaspoon whole cloves
- ✓ 1 thinly sliced orange
- ✓ 3-inch piece fresh ginger (unpeeled and well scrubbed)

Directions

- ✓ Cut large produce into chunks, and remove big seeds In a large saucepan, combine apple cider, cinnamon sticks, and whole cloves with orange and 3-inch piece fresh ginger (unpeeled and well scrubbed).

Orange Cinnamon Lassi

Lassi, an Indian yogurt-based drink, is refreshing and satisfying, especially with spicy dishes.
Servings: 4 | **Prep**: 10 mins | **Total time**: 10 mins

Ingredients

- ✓ 2 cups homemade yogurt or store-bought plain low-fat yogurt
- ✓ 2 tablespoons honey
- ✓ 2 cups whey ice cubes or plain ice cubes
- ✓ 1/4 teaspoon ground cinnamon, plus more for dusting
- ✓ 2 navel oranges

Directions

1. Place yogurt, honey, ice cubes, and cinnamon in a blender. Cut peel and pith from oranges. Working over a bowl, cut segments free of membranes. Transfer segments and juices in bowl to blender, and puree until mixture is smooth, about 1 minute.
2. Pour lassi into 4 chilled glasses; dust with cinnamon. Serve immediately.

Papaya Lassi

The ground cardamom in this refreshing papaya lassi brings out the flavor of the ripe fruit.

Serving: 4 | Prep Time: 5 mins | Total Time: 5 mins

Ingredients

- ✓ 2 cups chopped papaya (from 1 small peeled, seeded papaya)
- ✓ 1/2 cup ice
- ✓ 1 cup plain whole-milk yogurt
- ✓ 3 tablespoons sugar, or to taste
- ✓ Pinch of ground cardamom
- ✓ Pinch of coarse salt

Directions

- ✓ Combine papaya, ice, yogurt, sugar, cardamom, and salt in a blender; blend until smooth, 1 minute. Serve immediately.

Red Clover Vitamin Tonic

The blossoms of red clover are delicious, as any honeybee will demonstrate. This little wildflower makes a superlative tea, tasty and nutrient-rich by itself or combined with oats, nettle, violet, and mint, as in this tonic.

Serving: 1

Ingredients

- ✓ 3 teaspoons red-clover flowers/leaves
- ✓ 2 teaspoons oats, milky green tops (or oatstraw)
- ✓ 1 teaspoon nettle leaf
- ✓ 1 teaspoon violet leaves

✓ 2 teaspoons peppermint or spearmint

Directions

✓ Pour 1 quart boiling water over herbs; cover and steep for 15 to 20 minutes. Sweeten with honey if desired. Drink 2 to 3 cups daily for tonic benefits.

Simple Michelada

Tomato paste lends richness -- and a healthy serving of the antioxidant lycopene -- to this citrusy refresher. Kombucha, the popular fermented tea, delivers a satisfying fizz and gut-friendly probiotics.

Serving: 1

Ingredients

✓ Lime juice
✓ Sea salt, like Himalayan or Alaea
✓ 1 1/2 tablespoons tomato paste
✓ Ice
✓ 10 ounces kombucha

Directions

✓ Wet a glass rim with lime juice and dip into sea salt. Add 2 tablespoons lime juice and tomato paste and stir. Top with ice and kombucha. Stir to combine.

Spiced Pomegranate Punch

A spicy blend of pomegranate and orange juices and apple cider is served warm.

Yield: *Makes About 4 Cups*

Ingredients

✓ 5 pomegranates

- ✓ 1 cup apple cider
- ✓ 1/2 cinnamon stick
- ✓ 1 tablespoon thinly sliced fresh ginger
- ✓ 1/4 cup fresh orange juice, plus strips of orange zest for garnish

Directions

1. Cut pomegranates in half. Extract juice from seeds with a citrus juicer or reamer. Strain into a medium saucepan. (You should have about 2 1/2 cups juice.)
2. Add cider, 2 cups water, the cinnamon stick, and ginger. Cook over high heat until simmering, 5 to 6 minutes. Reduce heat; gently simmer 15 minutes. Skim any foam that rises to the surface.
3. Remove from heat. Discard cinnamon and ginger. Stir in orange juice. Serve warm, garnished with orange zest.

Spotted Cow

A quick root beer float is a great summer treat.
Yield: *Makes 4*

Ingredients

- ✓ 1 cup chocolate frozen yogurt
- ✓ 1 cup vanilla frozen yogurt
- ✓ 2 bottles (12 ounces each) chilled root beer

Directions

- ✓ Divide chocolate and vanilla frozen yogurt among four glasses. Carefully top with root beer.

Strawberry Banana Tofu Shake

Soft silken tofu provides the best results for this drink. If you only have firm or extra-firm silken tofu on hand, however, you can add as much as a quarter cup of extra soy milk to achieve the desired consistency. To reduce the fat, use the lite variety.

Servings: *4* | **Prep**: *10 mins* | **Total time**: *10 mins*

Ingredients

- ✓ 1 package (10 ounces) frozen, unsweetened strawberries, thawed
- ✓ 1 cup plain soymilk
- ✓ 1 small ripe banana, peeled and sliced
- ✓ 1/4 cup honey
- ✓ 1 package (12 ounces) silken soft tofu, drained
- ✓ 2 tablespoons fresh lemon juice
- ✓ Pinch of salt

Directions

1. In a blender, puree berries until smooth. Remove, and rinse blender.
2. Combine the remaining ingredients in the blender.
3. Puree until smooth and thoroughly mixed, scraping down sides with rubber spatula as necessary.
4. Divide among glasses and spoon strawberry puree on one side of each glass. Serve immediately or store in the refrigerator. If refrigerating, whisk to recombine just before serving.

The Hula Coola

Take canned sweetened cream of coconut, fresh pineapple, a big squirt of lemon, and some ice and blend. The result? The perfect Hawaiian cocktail. For a further tropical twist, add a paper umbrella.

Servings*: 4*

Ingredients

- ✓ 1/3 cup sweetened cream of coconut
- ✓ 2 cups cubed pineapple
- ✓ 1 tablespoon fresh lemon juice
- ✓ 1 cup ice cubes

Directions

- ✓ Put cream of coconut, pineapple, lemon juice, and ice into the pitcher of a blender, and blend for 15 seconds on high speed. (Always put the top on the container before processing.) Stop machine, and stir ingredients with a long wooden spoon. Blend for 15 seconds more on high speed.

Watermelon Nectar

This pink juice tastes as sweet and refreshing as a slice of the fruit -- with less mess.

Yield*: Makes About 5 1/2 Quarts*

Ingredients

- ✓ 1 seedless watermelon (about 12 pounds)

Directions

    ✓ Cut the flesh of a seedless watermelon into chunks, and puree them in batches in a blender. Strain the fruit through a sieve, and chill before serving.

Watermelon Punch and Bowl

Hollowed watermelon becomes a rustic serving bowl for a drink made with its juice, ensuring nothing goes to waste.

Servings: 10

Ingredients

    ✓ 1 oblong seedless watermelon (about 14 pounds)
    ✓ 3 cups seltzer

Directions

1. Cut top third off watermelon; trim bottom just enough to make a flat surface. Scoop out flesh.
2. Working in batches, puree watermelon in a food processor. Strain through a fine sieve; discard solids. (You should have about 9 cups juice.) Cover rind with plastic wrap. Refrigerate juice and rind until chilled, about 1 hour. Combine juice with seltzer; transfer to rind.

Conclusion

Thank you again for downloading this book!

I hope you enjoyed reading about my book!

Finally, if you enjoyed this book, please take the time to share your thoughts and post a review on Amazon. It'd be greatly appreciated!

Write me an honest review about the book – I truly value your opinion and thoughts and I will incorporate them into my next book, which is already underway.

Leave your review of my book here:

https://www.amazon.com/dp/ 1535277599

Thank you!

If you have any questions, feel free to contact at

contact@smallpassion.com

An Awesome Free Gift For You

Download Gift

http://www.smallpassion.com/awesome-gift

I want to say "Thank You" for buying my book so I've put together a few, awesome free gift for you **Tips and Techniques for Cooking Like a Chef & Delicious Desserts!** This gift is the perfect add-on this book and I know you'll love it. So click the link to go grab it.

Read more my book here:

http://www.amazon.com/author/anniekate
http://www.smallpassion.com/my-cookbooks

Annie Kate
Founder of www.SmallPassion.com

* * *